NEW BACH FLOWER BODY MAPS

NEW BACH FLOWER BODY MAPS

∾

TREATMENT

BY

TOPICAL

APPLICATION

∾

DIETMAR KRÄMER

TRANSLATED BY HANS-GEORG BAKKER

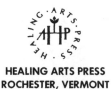

HEALING ARTS PRESS
ROCHESTER, VERMONT

Dedicated to the healer Heiner Müller,
who left us much too early.

ᄵ

Healing Arts Press
One Park Street
Rochester, Vermont 05767
www.InnerTraditions.com

Healing Arts Press is a division of Inner Traditions International

First Published in German under the title Neue Therapien mit Bach-Blüten 2
by Ansata-Verlag, Interlaken, Switzerland.

*Note to the reader: This book is intended as an informational guide. The remedies, approaches, and
techniques described herein are meant to supplement, and not to be a substitute for, professional
medical care or treatment. They should not be used to treat a serious ailment without prior
consultation with a qualified health care professional.*

Library of Congress Cataloging-in-Publication Data
Krämer, Dietmar.
[Neue Therapien mit Bach-Blüten 2. English]
New Bach flower body maps: treatment by topical application / Dietmar Krämer.
p.   cm.
Translation of: Neue Therapien mit Bach-Blüten 2.
Includes bibliographical references.
ISBN 978-0-89281-531-9
1. Flowers—Therapeutic use. 2. Transdermal medication. 3. Homeopathy—
Materia medica and therapeutics. I. Title
RX615.F55K73213   1996
615'.321—dc20   95-48845
CIP

Printed and bound in the United States
20 19 18 17

This book was typeset in Optima with Industria as the display typeface

CONTENTS

Acknowledgments

We would like to thank everybody who supported our work with Bach Flowers in a selfless way, especially Radha Bambeck for her helpful advice regarding arising problems; Cornelia Benzinger for her untiring assistance in the development of the skin zone topography; little Manuel for his invaluable comments about the changes of the aura, which actually gave us the idea for this work; and, finally, Mahavatar Babaji, without whose inspiration and always sensible help this project never could have been created.

Nothing can be acquired without knowledge; everything, however, can be achieved with a pure heart.

Babaji

FOREWORD

Body and soul are not two different parts, but two different ways to understand the same thing.

Albert Einstein

We live in a time of spiritual revolution, a time that encourages expansion of the mind and in turn creates an atmosphere conducive to global holistic research, medicine, and therapy. Holistic practices offer humankind the experience of spiritual manifestation. Through such practices ideals become reality; in a world of pollution, poisoning, decreasing quality of life, weakening of the immune system, and life-threatening events, these ideals made manifest produce a healing effect on flowers, animals, and people.

Due to humankind's interference with nature, we have entered a stage in which hundreds of thousands of people—hurt, sick, and without shelter—are challenged by forces and conditions seemingly out of their control. The further development of the flower therapies of Dr. Edward Bach by the authors of this book underscores the need to turn around the suffering that nature and humanity have entered into. Holistic treatments such as Bach Flower Therapy help to clear shock and negative emotional states and encourage the holistic healing of diseases and injuries.

The studies of science and spirituality prove that there is an abundance of intelligent forces and energies in creation that have not been recognized previously. Those forces are now being discovered and used in a beneficial and healing way in medicine and therapy.

Dina Rees, M.D.

Preface

With the publication of Dr. Edward Bach's *Heal Thyself* in 1931, a new era in the history of medicine began. Yet Edward Bach was to endure the fate of many other pioneers of genius: his healing method remained almost unknown for the next decades, despite the great accomplishments he and his successors were able to make. It was not until forty-eight years later that his books *Heal Thyself* and *The Twelve Healers,* along with Dr. F. J. Wheeler's *The Bach Remedies Repertory,* were published in German translation.

This book, entitled *New Bach Flower Body Maps,* is a kind of companion volume to *New Bach Flower Therapies* (Healing Arts Press, 1995). Why "new" therapies? The answer is simple: new therapeutic consequences, resulting from our practical work with the patient and an intuitive approach, have opened entirely new possibilities for Bach Flower Therapy in both diagnosis and application. A new treatment method, based on the ideas of the "tracks" and Bach Flower skin zones, has developed into an independent therapy. This new therapeutic concept is based on four principal elements, as described below.

CONSIDERATION OF THE RELATIONSHIP AMONG THE FLOWERS

Through the relationship of the flowers to each other (the tracks), it is possible to determine which flower covers the superficial side of a problem and which focuses more on the deeper cause. In this way a new hierarchy is created, one that will determine the therapy to follow. This hierarchy is especially helpful when a patient needs many flowers, a situation in which it can be difficult to find a starting point. Once the acute problems have diminished, it is possible with the help of this hierarchy to determine which of the deeper negative emotional states have led to the present complaints. It is then possible, if desired, to continue the therapy with the appropriate flowers to open up the mind.

ASTROLOGICAL DIAGNOSIS

Astrological psychology offers the opportunity to recognize deep emotional conflicts unknown to the patient. Thus it offers valuable diagnostic help, especially for children, who may be unable to recount a case history. The astrological diagnosis often provides the essential clue to the emotional reason for an illness.

In his book *The Twelve Healers of the Zodiac: The Astrology Handbook of the Bach Flower Therapies,* Peter Damian describes the use of twelve of the thirty-eight Bach Flowers in astrological diagnosis. The concept of the tracks allows us to incorporate thirty-two of the flowers in treating the emotional cause of illness or dis-ease. Five of the remaining six flowers deal specifically with external causes and influences and therefore are easy to recognize.

DIAGNOSIS THROUGH THE BACH FLOWER BODY MAPS

Similar to the reflex zones of the feet, every Bach Flower remedy is related to an area on the surface of the body. Negative moods lead to a change in the energetic structure of these places, which often is accompanied by pain and disturbing sensations in the physical body. Thus, it is possible to now obtain a flower diagnosis solely by consulting the body maps.

APPLICATION OF THE FLOWERS TO THE SKIN

It is possible to increase the effect of the flowers tremendously through application of Bach Flowers to the disturbed areas. Not only is it possible to improve negative emotional states much faster in this way than through oral tinctures, but the physical complaints often ease immediately as well. Bach Flower Therapy is thus not only a soul cleanser "to harmonize the psyche," as is often stated, but is also a therapy for the treatment of physical ailments.

This volume focuses on the use of the body maps. *New Bach Flower Therapies* focuses specifically on the tracks. These two volumes should be read and consulted together for a full understanding of our therapeutic concepts.

1
FOUNDATIONS

Treating the whole person and not just his illness was the leading idea fueling Dr. Edward Bach's life work. The focus of his work was the elimination of negative emotional states, which for him were the primary cause of any illness or state of dis-ease. At a lecture Dr. Bach stated: "Liberate your patient from one or multiple mood changes, as shown through this method of healing, and he will get better."[1]

Bach was able to observe how a person's emotional state changes in conjunction with disease, often even prior to the appearance of the first physical symptoms. He wrote: "During an illness the emotional state changes. . . . Anybody who watches carefully is able to perceive these changes often before—sometimes even a long time before—the appearance of the disease and thereby to prevent the appearance of complaints through early treatment."[2]

Although that statement indicates a possible prevention of disease, Bach in fact focused his work on the treatment of sick people, as many of his case studies show. His concern was to help people by means of a simple, harmless method, one that he thought would work better and would be easier to use in the treatment of incurable (at that time) diseases. This point has receded into the background in recent years: nowadays, Bach Flowers are seen in connection with the New Age and are viewed as a help in mastering inner conflicts, as a possible way to work on oneself, as a meditation aid, and as a method for inner cleansing or "soul hygiene." Edward Bach's original concern, however, was to find a plant-base alternative to the remedies he produced by pathological intestinal bacteria. With the bacterial remedies, given by injection, he was able to ease arthritis pains and strong headaches, an unparalleled accomplishment for medicine in those days. His homeopathic processing of those preparations, known as Bach nosodes, made him a place in the history of homeopathy. The preparations became a great success and gave Edward Bach the reputation of a second Hahnemann.

It is almost unthinkable that he would have given up those useful therapies to find a healing method that would simply increase well-being and bring about emotional harmony. His goal was to eliminate the emotional causes of disease, and to thereby make their physical consequences vanish. To achieve that goal he used his remedies not only internally; he also applied them externally in the form of compresses or liniments on the affected area. He wrote: "For pain, stiffness, inflammation, or any kind of local ailments one should also use a lotion. A few drops from the stock bottle are put into a bowl of water and a piece of cloth is soaked in it and applied to the affected areas. If necessary one can rewet the cloth again and again."[3]

One example should explain Bach's procedure:

> Shortly after he discovered the healing potential of Vervain, Bach was called to a patient who had slipped on the sidewalk and had sprained his ankle. When Bach arrived at 10 P.M. the man's ankle was vastly swollen, which caused him a great deal of pain.
>
> The patient was a strongly built, extremely impatient man of nearly fifty years. He thought it would take about three weeks for his injury to heal, and he was convinced that he could not afford such a long break from his job. He was vital and enthusiastic about things and had the tendency to exhaust himself with his professional life. It was difficult for him to relax. His strong will kept him going even when he ought to have taken a rest.
>
> The patient's restlessness called for the application of the Impatiens remedy; his tendency toward inner tension and his enthusiasm for work, as well as his urge for activity, demanded treatment with Vervain.
>
> Two or three drops of each remedy were added to a bowl of warm water. A compress soaked in the liquid was wrapped around the patient's ankle, and he was instructed to rewet the compress every time it became dry.
>
> By the next day the patient was able to go about his work, and in the evening of the same day he was able to walk normally again. He was even seen stamping his affected foot, saying: "It can't be true that I really sprained my ankle."[4]

Edward Bach also treated more serious illnesses, such as asthma, arthritis, and leukemia, in the same way, as Nora Weeks's biography of him shows. (See Further Reading for Weeks's book and others related to the Bach system.)

Edward Bach viewed his method of treatment as a further development of homeopathy. In a speech in which Bach talked about homeopathy, he said about its founder: "Hahnemann made a great advance and carried us a long way along the road, but he had only the length of one life in which to work, and it is for us to continue his research where he left off: to add more to the structure of perfect healing of which he laid the foundation and so worthily began the building."[5]

This book and *New Bach Flower Therapies* (Healing Arts Press, 1995) should be considered a continuation of Edward Bach's work. Originating out of our practical work and intuitive exploration of this method, these companion volumes represent an addition to and expansion of the knowledge about the flowers that Bach specified as the "flowers of higher order." Over the last fifty years, this kind of development has been rare in the field of Bach Flower Therapies, while in homeopathy much progress and expansion of knowledge has been achieved in the same time period. We do not question the principles formulated by Dr. Bach, nor do we intend to contradict his teachings in any way. Rather we want to build on his findings, to gain new knowledge and to add new pieces to the mosaic.

We are strongly convinced that this would be the intention of Edward Bach, who certainly did not want to create dogma out of his work. In one of his letters Bach wrote about the assignment of zodiac signs, planets, and physical symptoms to the flowers: "However, it seems to be my task to give general principles, which can help people like you who possess detailed knowledge to discover a great truth. Therefore, I do not want to be affiliated with anything dogmatic, as long as one is not absolutely certain."[6]

In another letter he wrote: "All true knowledge originates out of our inner self, in quiet communication with our soul. Doctrines and civilizations have exploited us from our stillness, have taken away from us this knowledge: We know everything deep in ourselves. We were made to believe that we need to be instructed, and our own spiritual self was suppressed."[7]

His method ought to be as simple as possible, free of any detailed medical knowledge and intellectual ballast: "I want to make it that easy: If I am hungry I go into the garden and pick a salad. If I am afraid, I take a dose of Mimulus."[8]

The therapy with the Bach Flower skin zones makes treatment even easier than that: The required remedy can be read directly from the body, simply by recognizing the localization of the complaints. A search for the right flower among several flowers found by means of an interview or by interpretation of the symptoms given through the language of the body is no longer necessary. This simplification offers the possibility of an even more direct and effective treatment of physical ailments, as was Edward Bach's original intention.

Edward Bach was a sensitive—when he put a leaf of a flower on his tongue, he was able to "feel" the symptoms that flower would be able to cure. His classification of flower remedies and symptoms makes it possible for everybody to heal with his established remedy tables. We hold the similar intention of offering a therapy developed in a way that anyone can work with it. For people who are sensitives, this therapy offers the possibility of applying their abilities in a more systematic way.

DISCOVERY OF BACH FLOWER SKIN ZONES

Bach Flower Therapy with skin zones was actually initiated by the sensitive people who came into our office. Due to their abilities to see the aura, they often produced important clues about the emotional state of a patient they observed without the patient being aware of such a "diagnosis." We were especially interested in their help with patients who did not seem to respond to treatment. The phenomena that they described in those therapy-resistant cases were almost always the same: The aura of therapy-resistant patients showed very dark colors—often a combination of dark red, dark brown, and black—and there were holes in the aura.

According to the literature and documentation concerning the aura, dark colors start to appear with emotional states of hate and bitterness. Questioned about this, the individuals often answered that there was a person in their lives who had induced so much pain that they still were not able to forgive, even though the incident had happened many years before. Other patients felt they had not been fairly treated or perceived themselves as victims of fate. Some of those people had resigned internally and given up on themselves. With these people, the states of Willow and Wild Rose respectively were indeed confirmed as the strongest therapeutic obstacles.

The observed holes in the aura at first did not make much sense to us. Only years later did we apply some drops of Willow as a test to the place on the body corresponding to the hole in the aura of a person who had given us the impression that she was embittered. Immediately after application of the flower remedy she told us that she was able to see everything more clearly, as if somebody had turned on a light.

Several months later we started our first specific trial: A fifty-year-old patient came to the office with pain in her sacrum and her right hip. Her family doctor had treated her with injections and low-voltage treatments without any success. First, we gave her a few drops of Pine on her sacrum and waited ten minutes for a reaction. Immediately the patient reported a feeling of relief, which expanded into her entire back. This was followed by a pulling sensation, radiating from her back to the solar plexus in the front and further into her lungs. A long-standing feeling of pressure in her solar plexus subsided and gave way to a feeling of relief.

Next, we applied a few drops of Vervain to her throat in the area of the thyroid. The patient had not complained about any pain in that area, but we had observed major changes in the aura at that point. Shortly afterward she told us that her head felt much lighter and her thoughts had become freer. Throughout the last weeks she had had a rather dull sensation that was almost like a feeling of fog in front of her eyes. That also completely disappeared.

After a few more minutes we massaged a few drops of Wild Oat into the painful area on her right hip. The pain immediately eased, and only a minimal pressure remained. Along with it, a feeling of rigidity also disappeared from her lower abdomen. Ten minutes later the patient got up from the table pain free.

The Kirlian photographs taken before and after the treatment show the enormous change in the patient's energy flow (see page 6). The fact that the feet became visible in the second picture indicates that the energetic blockage in the center of the body had dissolved. The radiation of energy around the hands—signs of a hormonal imbalance—also had normalized. We are absolutely convinced that feelings of guilt can trigger hormonal disturbances in the organs of the lower abdomen. Most likely, guilt feelings are even the main cause for these disturbances. This particular patient returned for a follow-up visit a week later and had no further complaints.

Later on we were able to establish other Bach Flower skin zones in a similar fashion. In being preoccupied with changes in the aura we became so sensitive that it was possible for us to eventually feel the disturbances of others in our own bodies when they would come close to us. For example, the right arm would feel a burning sensation without any apparent reason. We then would concentrate our minds on this particular area and try to understand what the body wanted to tell us by the burning pain. Afterward, we would apply a few drops of the suspected flower remedy—in that case Wild Rose—to the area. When we chose the right one, the pain would instantly subside. This particular patient who had caused the sensation in us also needed this flower. While the patient may have experienced pain at the same spot on his body, he certainly had a corresponding hole in his aura.

My own (Dietmar's) sensitivity finally became so strong that I was able to feel such a transmission even when I was in a different room. Through intensive work with the aura and the Bach Flower experiments, my colleague (Helmut) gained the ability to actually see the aura. In this way we often were able to diagnose patients as they entered our office.

In the same way that we were able to feel the negative states of mind of other people relative to corresponding skin areas, we were eventually able to feel our own. When we felt anger, the Holly skin area started to tingle. If we reacted impatiently in a certain situation, the head started to itch in an unpleasant way in the Impatiens area. (Interestingly, many people scratch themselves on this spot when they feel restless.) When we gave in too easily,

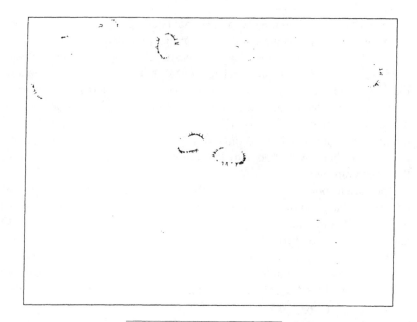

Kirlian photograph before Bach Flower treatment.

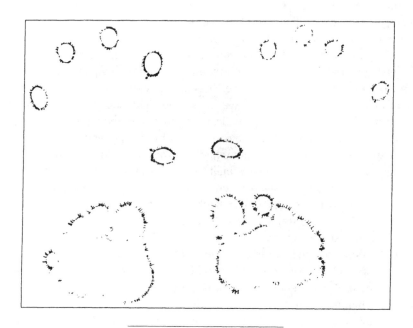

Kirlian photograph after Bach Flower treatment.

we felt pressure at the chest. From different sensations such as tingling, tickling, itching, burning, pressure, and so forth, we obtained information about the quality of the emotions embodied in the flowers.

In this way we also learned that negative emotions produce changes not only in the color of the aura but also in its shape. Anger creates not only dark red to black colors but also an indentation in the area of the liver, for example. The size is dependent on the intensity of the emotion; it creates either a small dent or a hole. When the person has calmed down, the shape of the aura normalizes. Chronic anger creates lasting changes, however, and will create physical complaints in corresponding body areas.

The assignment of Bach Flowers to certain skin areas according to the manifestation of negative emotions in the body corresponds only partially to what is already known through the language of the organs. A large number of areas cannot be explained in that way and obviously follow their own rules. For example, the Bach Flower skin zones show that the attribution of fear to the kidneys is not complete; the skin zones show that the left kidney corresponds to a feeling of inner impurity. The left kidney not only purifies the body and excretes its waste, but also, as stated in the Chinese acupuncture teachings, cleans the body of impure energy, which after being absorbed with the food will end up in the kidney through the so-called lower heater. A connection with the Crab Apple flower is therefore very plausible.

Why, however, the left kidney corresponds especially to this feeling of impurity while the right one has a much closer connection to fear cannot easily be explained in the context of the language of the organs. (See *New Bach Flower Therapies* for more information on the language of the organs.) It is possible that the kidneys follow the same energetic principle as the brain, the left side corresponding to the active principle (yang) and recognized as the place of intellect, and the right side embodying the passive principle (yin) and acknowledged as the place of emotions.

CHANGES IN THE AURA AFTER APPLICATION TO THE SKIN

Rubbing some drops of the appropriate flower into an area corresponding to a hole in the aura will cause the following reactions to happen within minutes:

First, the aura's colors on the edge of the hole will mix with each other. The new blend of colors mostly corresponds to the well-known color mixes, meaning blue and yellow will make green, red and blue will create violet, and so forth. Alterations are possible, however. The edge of this area, where the flower drops do not moisten the skin, becomes visible as a thin interrupted line of mixed colors.

Next, at the place where the hole is the thinnest, a sticky, mostly violet mass is formed that in its consistency is more dense than the surrounding aura. Just like a stream of lava, it will flow into the hole and slowly fill it up.

After the hole is completely covered, a skinlike surface is formed; this surface covers the whole area like a tarp and protects it from external influences. This surface will show a somewhat lighter color. The spot with its tone of color will stay visible until the negative emotion is completely cleared from consciousness, which sometimes can take from several weeks to a few months. Only then will it adopt the same color as the surrounding aura.

Often a single application of the flowers is not effective. Depending on the degree of the emotional conflict, the hole can form again after hours or days. If the wrong flower is applied to the skin at an area of change in the aura, the colors also will mix. However, after a few seconds this mix will again change and the original status will be regained.

For each patient one flower exists that matches that person quite well and will show the same effect on each area as the flowers designated specifically for those areas. Similar to the constitutional remedy in homeopathy, that flower corresponds to the real character of the individual and is called a type remedy. It can be quite difficult to find, and it does not always correspond to the most prominent character trait of the person. Often, though, it will make itself known during the course of therapy. For that reason, the treatment with the appropriate flowers for the skin areas is much easier and leads to a more positive outcome than trial and error with possible type remedies. During a proper Bach Flower treatment this type remedy will be given anyway to dissipate the underlying negative emotion.

Due to his sensitivity, Edward Bach was able to find the most suitable flower remedy on the first trial. The same successes Dr. Bach had in his treatment of physical symptoms will be encouraged by the use of the body maps.

EFFECT ON THE BODY AND THE PSYCHE

If the hole in the aura closes up and stays closed for some time, one of the following reactions will occur:

    ∾ The complaints—physical or emotional—will disappear within seconds, especially in sensitive patients, who sometimes can permanently eliminate all of their physical symptoms through the use of compresses and liniments. Additional therapy with other more physically oriented naturopathic treatments is usually not required for those patients. Here are two examples:

A twenty-seven-year-old female patient felt intense pain in her left lower abdomen. Since she had suffered from infections of her ovaries, she was worried that she might be unable to have more children. After Rock Rose was rubbbed into the affected area, her pain subsided within seconds and did not recur.

A sixty-year-old female patient told us that for weeks she had been aggressive for no apparent reason. Sometimes she even would yell at people without knowing why. She said that this behavior was absolutely new for her and her change in character worried her very much. She also had felt quite dull recently and had the feeling of being mentally "far away." Three drops of Holly were rubbed into a spot at the back of her head. For the closing of her aura she received a drop of Centaury on her tongue. Shortly afterward she felt absolutely normal again. Two years later, this change in character has never recurred.

- ∾ The patient will not feel an immediate effect, but through a regular application of the flowers the complaints will slowly dissolve within days or weeks.
- ∾ The patient will not feel any relief, even after continuous applications. The illness is already so advanced, or has penetrated so far into the organic-physiologic level, that impulses from the emotional body are not strong enough to eliminate the damage. In this case the Bach Flowers will hasten the effects of other healing methods such as homeopathy, acupuncture, and neuromuscular therapy, while continuing to help in the elimination of the emotional causes of illness.

In some cases the hole in the aura closes up for only a short time, only to open again just a few minutes later. The physical symptoms also do not resolve, even after repeated applications. This could be caused by one of the following reasons:

- ∾ The patient is lacking the inner readiness to change or to let go of the negative emotions underlying his condition. In such cases the success of Bach Flowers is minimal.
- ∾ The energetic disturbance is located somewhere else. The actual "center" is silent, meaning it does not create any complaints.

Since in most such cases we deal with a zone of the same flower or with a corresponding flower, it is possible to find the appropriate flower for the condition even without sensitive abilities by using the tracks described in *New Bach Flower Therapies*. The positive reactions—whether the complaints get better immediately or after several applications—are often accompanied by subjective perceptions that occur immediately after application of the flower to the skin. The following sensations might be observed:

- A feeling of relief, as if a heavy weight had been taken off
- Feeling looser and more relaxed inside
- A sensation of seeing everything more brightly and clearly
- A feeling of rest and relaxation; the muscle tone changes, facial muscles start to relax, and sometimes a smile appears
- A feeling of being more awake and clear, especially with the applications of Olive and Wild Rose.

In some cases—especially when there are no physical symptoms in a particular area—reactions occur that reveal energetic blockages due to negative emotions and, therefore, have somewhat the character of a therapeutic experience. Some examples:

A twenty-seven-year-old female patient was tormented by strong feelings of guilt and self blame. After Pine was rubbed onto her sacrum, she experienced the following reactions: First, she had an intense feeling of warmth in the treated area. That was followed by a sensation of energy flowing toward the front, into the genital area, and finally up into the Pine zone, around the area of the solar plexus. A feeling of restlessness then occurred in her head, solely on the left side, which came and went in waves. The sensation of heat became more and more intense and spread out sideways. Next, she felt the heat in her face just above the left cheek (zygoma), and at the same time the restless feeling in her head disappeared. The sensation on her sacrum increased to a burning heat, and she grew increasingly tired. At the end of the session she was completely exhausted.

After a rubdown with Wild Rose on his right arm, a young man reported feeling as if a valve had opened up that allowed all the negative energy to escape from him. This reaction happened within seconds. Afterward he felt a tremendous inner and outer relief, as if a negative force had been taken off him. A year later he told me that the effects of the session were lasting, and that he never again felt as dull as he did prior to the treatment.

In these examples only the reactions to the flowers specific to the particular zones were being observed. If the wrong flower was applied to a disturbed area, no spontaneous positive reaction would be observed except for a sensation of coldness, which is caused by evaporation. Positive results can occur, however, if a flower that is well suited to the patient but does not match the particular zone is given over an extended period. This "type remedy," applied anywhere on the body, will produce the same results in the aura as the flower specific to the zone. However, the sensations usually are not as intense as the ones felt with the application of a matching flower to the area needing treatment, and the healing progresses more slowly.

There are some exceptions in which *only* the type remedy creates the breakthrough, but that reaction does not occur very often. Here is an example of the application of the type remedy:

> A sixty-three-year-old female patient suffered from a hand-size fungal infection on her right upper thigh in the Agrimony zone. The skin was very red and crusted over. Because the common ointments against fungus had failed and the infection was expanding, her family doctor ordered a cortisone ointment, but she did not want such an intensive therapy and was seeking a gentler healing method. Rather than administering the flower that corresponded to the zone, her type remedy was applied to the aggravated skin zone. Immediately after receiving several drops of the Chicory flower, the redness began to fade. The woman was instructed to rub the skin zone twice a day with undiluted Chicory from the stock bottle.
>
> During the following weeks the skin slowly softened, though the redness persisted. When the dried skin was finally gone, the redness also disappeared.

This reaction shows that the body needed the inflammation to fight the fungus. Only after the fungus was completely subdued was the inflammation, visible as redness, able to disappear, because it was no longer necessary. Rather than allowing for a true healing response, the cortisone treatment would have simply suppressed the inflammation, masking the symptoms but allowing the imbalance to stay lodged in the body. The possible consequences of such an approach are well known in naturopathic medicine.

After four weeks of treatment, the patient's skin rash was completely healed.

2
FINDING THE SKIN ZONES

ACTIVE ZONES

Active zones are defined as body areas that express disturbance through a particular sensation or physical symptom, such as:

- Localized pain
- Disturbing sensations such as tingling or itching
- Sensitivity to pressure
- Skin rashes
- Any kind of localized changes of the skin.

The changes noticeable at the skin level (the active zones) make it possible to use the body maps to determine which flower is needed to treat a given complaint.

SILENT ZONES

Silent zones are defined as areas of the body that are disturbed but do not manifest physical changes of any kind. Silent zones can be determined through recognizing changes in the patient's aura. These silent zones can develop for several reasons:

1. The disturbance is based on an emotional conflict that has not yet expressed itself physically. By treating the area of the body directly

underneath the auric change with the flower indicated by the body maps, the conflict can be dissolved much faster than by taking the flower orally.

2. The disturbance manifests itself in an area different from the one directly underneath the auric change, meaning that the actual "center" of the disturbance is silent. Usually this silent zone belongs to the same flower as the one indicated by the auric change, though sometimes a different flower can be considered based on the use of the tracks (see *New Bach Flower Therapies*). In extremely rare cases, the complaint appears in a spot that is completely unrelated to the actual disturbance. In such instances the sensitive diagnosis can play an important role. Another possibility for therapy is to try the zones of the flowers that, following the interview, match most closely the character of the individual.

3. The disturbance can be traced to an emotional conflict in the past that has already been solved but about which outdated information remains at that particular area of the body. Only after that information has been erased from the memory of the cells is it possible to completely dissolve the negative emotion.

In some cases silent zones are anatomically conspicuous, and the body surface itself offers clues. In those areas one might find a birthmark, more body hair, a decrease of hair compared with the surrounding areas, or conspicuous redness or paleness of the skin.

The phenomenon of the silent zones shows us that changing one's consciousness is not in itself sufficient to solve an emotional problem. Negative emotions can remain present as misinformation on the energetic level. For this reason, silent zones represent a much bigger block in therapy than active zones, and treatment of the silent zones will bring the greatest success in the course of a Bach Flower treatment.

DETECTION OF SILENT ZONES

Physical Complaints

If the treatment of an active zone is unsuccessful, it should be suspected that the main energetic disturbance is located in a different zone. In that case it is recommended to proceed in the following way, especially if there is no sensitive diagnosis for clarification.

First, try to obtain a positive reaction by treating further zones of the same flower. According to our observations, the zones on the trunk are the most highly reactive, so it is suggested that the appropriate zones on the trunk be treated with the same flower remedy specified for the active zone.

Any abatement in the symptoms indicates that the treated area is the right one. Know that true healing takes time; one should not expect miracles right away. If the diagnosis is the right one, however, results should be seen after a few applications.

If no improvement can be seen, the zones appropriate to companion flowers as found through the tracks should be treated, especially the zones on the trunk (see *New Bach Flower Therapies,* and in this book see "Diagnosis with the Tracks," page 15). If there is still no positive result, one should use the flower that emerged as most prominent in the interview, from the more traditional assessment techniques of organ language (see *New Bach Flower Therapies*) and the emotional symptoms given in the Bach profiles. Apply this flower to its zones as shown by the body maps. If this approach still does not prove to be successful, personal and possibly subconscious blocks to therapy should be considered. It may be that the person does not really want to get well because the illness offers certain advantages. Perhaps, due to many earlier failures, the patient does not really believe that recovery is possible. In this case, the Gorse skin zone in the area of the left shoulder (see page 109) will be quite sensitive to pressure. Treatment at this particular spot, supported by the oral ingestion of Gorse —preferably in a water solution—is certainly a good idea.

In many cases, treatment of the sacrum with Pine essence can dissolve blocks to therapy by restoring hormonal regulation. Feelings of guilt often remain subliminal or are regarded as normal due to a puritanical religious education. Due to their localization on the body—at the solar plexus, the back of the head, and especially at the sacrum—guilt feelings are capable of disturbing the entire endocrine and energetic regulation of the body. The sacrum is also the reflex zone of the reproductive organs, which produce hormones important to balanced emotional functioning. For this reason, Pine zones have a priority in the treatment if they are identified as necessary.

In cases of complaints that are not precisely localized, emotional symptoms should be used to distinguish the appropriate flower therapy. If, for example, a hypochondriac patient complains about chest pain, the Heather zone around the heart should be considered (see page 114). If a patient suffers a bad case of homesickness, the Honeysuckle zone should be treated.

Finally, we can say that the treatment of active zones offers success in most cases, provided that the effect of the flowers is sufficient to heal the respective physical symptoms. If massive organic disturbances are already present, the flowers are used mainly as a support for other forms of therapy.

Emotional Problems

When working with emotional problems, we use the flowers externally only at the beginning of the treatment. To treat emotional problems through the skin zones, it is recommended to start with the particular flower that embodies the strongest decompensation state.* If the specific skin zones to which the flower should be applied cannot be determined by sight, the flower is used on all the appropriate skin zones on the trunk and possibly the head. If more than one decompensation flower is indicated, a total of three flowers could be applied simultaneously. Once the decompensation state is remedied, the flower will show very good effects through its internal use and will no longer require support through its skin zones.

The application of the flowers to the skin zones is especially beneficial for severe moodiness and internal conflicts, which may be resistant to the internal ingestion of the flower drops. For more external problems such as deadlines or performance anxieties, or for shock that comes from unexpected events, the internal use of the flowers is most often sufficient.

Diagnosis with the Tracks

If the treatment of a skin zone with its corresponding flower has been unsuccessful, it is quite possible that the patient has already entered the compensation or decompensation state. In this case, use of the more superficial flower on its skin zone will bring the desired success.† Here is an example:

> A middle-aged female patient complained about a headache. After rubbing Rock Water into the affected area, she felt no change in her pain. However, after the application of Crab Apple to its corresponding zone in the neck area, the pain instantly subsided. Obviously, the patient had

---

* For a thorough understanding of the relationships of the flowers to each other; the successive states of communication, compensation, and decompensation; and the inner and outer (or superficial) flower designations, read *New Bach Flower Therapies,* chapter 2, "A New Classification of the Flowers."

† When the communication state is not balanced, the condition becomes progressively deeper rooted, leading to the compensation and finally to the decompensation states. While it seems that the communication flower would be considered the superficial flower, it is actually the compensation and decompensation states that one notices at the surface. For that reason, these flowers are considered superficial in relationship to the communication flower.

already entered the state of decompensation; otherwise, she would have shown a positive reaction to Rock Water.

At this point we want to emphasize again that the treatment through the skin zones is only one aspect of Bach Flower therapy. Every treatment begins with an in-depth interview, which clarifies the actual complaints and the compensation or decompensation state at the very beginning of the session. In addition to the external application, the flowers considered for treatment will also be given internally.

The application of the entire group of flowers of one track should be avoided, since this can cause a severe reaction that cannot be explained solely through the effect of the flowers. However, under certain circumstances it *is* possible to specifically use the entire track to potentiate the effect of the flowers, although certain rules have to be followed.

If all three flowers of a track are indicated and the symptoms occur in an area designated to the communication flower, the following route of action is recommended. First, the communication and decompensation flowers are given orally, while simultaneously the communication flower is applied externally. Once the decompensation state is dissolved, the compensation flower alone is given orally, while external application of the communication flower is continued. For example, assume that the patient complains about chest pain in the area of the Centaury zone (see page 58), and simultaneously mentions feelings of guilt. Centaury and Pine are given orally, and Centaury is also applied in the form of compresses or salves to the painful area. (Centaury, Holly, and Pine comprise one track.) If the therapy does not progress as anticipated, Pine can also be applied externally to the corresponding zones. In this case, the zone in the solar plexus area (see page 167) should be considered first, since it is closest in proximity to the main physical complaint.

Once the feeling of guilt has subsided, Holly is given orally; at this point the oral application of Pine is stopped. If the physical symptoms have not completely ceased, Centaury can still be applied externally. Otherwise, the oral application will be sufficient.

DIAGNOSIS THROUGH THE AURA

The diagnosis of the energy body by those who can see and feel the aura is so far the only known objective method for determining which Bach Flower corresponds to a specific zone on the skin. A reading of the aura shows which flowers an individual needs by indicating where they are needed. (See Appendix II for more on the aura.) With the help of the aura it is possible to uncover subconscious emotional conflicts and latent physical disturbances; the aura reveals connections between negative emotions and physical complaints in a direct way. Often entire tracks become visible, as, for example, for the combination of asthma (Centaury zone), gallstones (Holly zone), and gastric ulcers (Pine zone).

For this reason, study of the auric diagnostic method is very beneficial, particularly since the ability to feel and see the aura unknowingly exists in many people. Time and again during seminars and lectures we have found that, after an appropriate introduction, approximately two-thirds of the participants were able to feel auras without previously being aware of this ability.

People who can feel the phenomenon of the aura with their hands can be divided into two groups. The first group can sense the edges of the aura and thereby find the bulged and indented areas. The other group can feel changes in the aura; they feel elevations as a heat sensation on the skin and they feel holes as intense cold sensations. Other phenomena are perceived as tingling sensations.

Sensitivity to the aura and the ability to read auric changes develops and strengthens with training and practice. Auric reading is a very helpful tool in using the Bach Flowers.

3

THE PRACTICE OF BACH FLOWER SKIN ZONE THERAPY

The only criteria for treatment with Bach Flower remedies on the skin zones is the willingness of the patient to change. Therefore, an interview and assessment, as explained in *New Bach Flower Therapies,* is necessary. In a seemingly obvious diagnosis from the skin zones, where an interview would be unnecessary, one should at least offer an explanation about the effect of the flowers prior to their application to the skin. A treatment without the knowledge and consent of the individual represents a violation of the individual's free will and can lead to intense reactions if he or she is not willing to change on the emotional level. One should not use the simple therapeutic tool of the Bach Flowers unethically.

For acute problems it is sufficient to explain the connection between physical symptoms and emotional causes in a few words, and to receive consent for the treatment.

INDICATIONS FOR TREATMENT

Physical Complaints

The treatment of physical ailments of every kind represents the main area of indication of Bach Flowers. Pain is a warning sign from the body and can be treated only if its origin is known. However, something like acute appendicitis can be fatally dangerous when the appendix ruptures, and consequently represents a medical emergency. It is evident from the literature that Edward Bach treated serious diseases almost solely with Bach Flowers. However, as a doctor he knew what he was doing and was able to use other methods of treatment in an emergency if the patient did not respond to the flowers. It is extremely important that a naturopathic physician or a doctor investigate acute bodily symptoms of pain. We do not recommend self-diagnosis of acute conditions.

It is possible to use Bach Flowers as an accompaniment to medical or naturopathic therapy, or for minor complaints, such as:

- Tension headaches due to overwork or lack of sleep
- Tension and tightness along the spine, for example, neck pain or tightness of the shoulders
- Complaints due to exhaustion
- Sore muscles
- Minor injuries, bruises, and abrasions
- Physical effects of emotional states, for example, gallbladder pain during anger, abdominal pressure during arguments, itching in uncomfortable situations, and so forth
- Impurities of the skin and acne
- Harmless rashes such as nervous urticaria (redness, hives, and itching), sunburn and sun allergies, minor burns, and so forth (The formation of pus or other discharge requires consultation with a physician or naturopath.)
- Simple colds, congestion, and coughs
- Chronic fatigue states with no apparent underlying illness
- Tingling and other forms of disturbance in one's overall skin sensitivity.

The entire list of indications for treatment through the skin zones is described in *New Bach Flower Therapies*.

Emotional Complaints

The treatment of emotional problems through the Bach Flower skin zones represents the most direct method of psychotherapy available. The negative emotions are treated in the exact area in which they show themselves in the soul body—the aura—and where they will make themselves noticeable in the form of physical symptoms if they remain unresolved. Negative emotions will vanish much faster with this method than with the oral application of drops. Sometimes they disappear within seconds. Overall, therapy with the Bach Flower skin zones advances much faster.

In some cases we noticed that treatment of the skin zones was successful within a short period of time, while previous oral application of the same flower had been without any effect over weeks or even months. Negative emotions are seemingly stored in the body's cells; in cases of deep conflict, the emotions can be released only if the right information is brought to the exact spot where the emotions are located inside the body. The success of color radiation of acupuncture points seems to confirm this theory. Recent studies suggest that cells indeed possess real memory. As mentioned earlier, the emotional state often changes prior to the occurrence of the first physical symptoms of disease. When illness finally happens, it usually manifests itself in the skin zones associated with the negative emotional state as indicated by the aura. Consequently, in cases of intense emotional change it is possible to apply the flowers to those areas to prevent the organic effect of an emotional disturbance. It should be remembered that deep-seated emotional conflicts need more time to be completely resolved.

APPLICATIONS

Compresses

Next to rubbing flowers into the skin directly from the stock bottle, compresses are the most effective form of application. Since the former method is often not recommended for reasons discussed on page 22, compresses are preferred for intense complaints or persistent problems.

To prepare a compress, two drops of the appropriate flower are added to half a glass of water. A piece of cloth is soaked in this mixture. If more than one flower is used, a solution is made for each. If the constitutional or type remedy is known, it can be mixed into a solution to potentiate its effects.

The wet towels stay on the skin zones for ten minutes. Depending on the intensity of the complaints, the compresses should be used one to three times a day, and more frequently for extreme complaints.

Creams

The use of flowers in the form of a cream represents the easiest application method. Up to three flowers can be combined in a cream mixture. Although when prepared in this way the flowers are applied together to the corresponding zones, the effect is the same as with the use of different creams containing only one flower each. The cream base will penetrate the skin very slowly, forming a film on the skin that will last a long while. We have had very good results with collagen creams, which are quite skin friendly and not as sticky as other creams, such as those with a lanolin base.

To prepare the flower cream, two drops of each flower are combined in

10 g of a cream base. The skin zones are treated two to three times a day. For strong complaints, a more frequent application is possible.

Although this application method is much easier than the compresses, the effect is less dramatic. In cases of very developed disturbances, intense pain, or therapy-resistant complaints, compresses should be used first. The same is recommended for cases in which creams have little or no effect. Once a significant improvement or elimination of the symptoms has been effected, further treatment with creams will be sufficient.

Tinctures

For the treatment of zones on the head that are covered by hair, the application of a tincture is recommended. The tincture is mixed in the same dilution as the solution prepared for internal use: one drop of the flower to 10 cc of liquid. The best solvent is distilled water, which guarantees a long shelf life. Alcohol should be avoided, as it can irritate the skin in cases of continuous use. To make application easier, pipettes instead of droppers are recommended.

Lotions

Another form of application is a lotion application; however, lotion application is only beneficial if the constitutional or type remedy is known. Since the type remedy is appropriate for all disturbed body zones, it is beneficial to make a lotion and apply it daily to the whole body—after showering, for example. In this way, the disturbed skin zones can be treated simultaneously without knowing them specifically. The only condition regarding lotion application is that the flower be the constitutional remedy; otherwise the desired effect will not occur.

The only criterion known to date that will determine the individual flower or type remedy with absolute certainty is that the remedy have a positive effect on every skin zone. Since only diagnostically sensitive people can unequivocally determine a patient's type remedy, use of the body maps and application of the corresponding flowers to the skin zones is the easiest and safest method for the nonsensitive user. Over time, the few flowers that represent one's deepest negative emotions will become quite prominent. It is likely that one of those flowers will also be the correct constitutional remedy.*

---

* The "shortcut" of the type remedy has its drawbacks, as treatment via several flowers that are found by interview, through the language of the organs, or through the disturbed skin zones, can bring enormous insight about the inner causes of the patient's present problems.

Through therapeutic work with the skin zones, patients will understand the connection between negative emotional states and physical symptoms. As a result of the internal use of the Bach Flowers, patients become aware of their interaction with the environment and responses to daily events. During the course of the treatment they learn to overcome or prevent problems and illnesses by altering their own attitudes and behaviors. Thus they are in a position to understand and experience fully the lesson that life offers to them in each moment. This realization is the true meaning of the phrase "mind expansion."

POSSIBLE REACTIONS FOR THE PRACTITIONER

To study the flowers' effects on the aura and the resulting physical and emotional reactions, and also to draw the body maps, we first applied undiluted drops from the stock bottle to the client's body. Our experiences showed us that, under certain circumstances, a strong reaction can occur for the practitioner. This reaction is evidently caused by the transformation of the practitioner's physical and emotional symptoms which, if not registered and acted upon accordingly, can last for days or in some cases even for weeks.

On the other hand, applying the drops directly from the stock bottle to oneself is relatively harmless. The only risk in doing this is a later recurrence of the symptoms in a stronger form or a relocation of the symptoms to another area of the body, either of which will disappear after rubbing in the appropriate flower. This, however, can be completely avoided by treating the area with compresses for two weeks prior to using the rubdowns.

Based on our experience we find it necessary to strongly warn against a direct application of the undiluted flower remedies by a therapist onto a patient. We recommend the application of the flowers in the form of compresses or salves, which also will show fast results. It is interesting to note that, according to the literature available to us, Edward Bach never used the flowers in a pure form but always diluted them. Even in the case of acute injuries, he applied them externally only in the form of compresses, baths, sponge rubbings, or lotions. The only exception to this practice was in the case of unconscious people, to whom Dr. Bach gave the Rescue Remedy in its undiluted form.

4
OTHER APPLICATIONS

INDICATIONS THAT DIFFER FROM THE TOPOGRAPHY

If external influences have caused local disturbances, the external flowers should be used.* Since these flowers directly address the situational cause of the complaint, they act more intensely and longer than the designated flowers of the injured zones. The diagnosis of which flower remedy to use must be made according to the nature of the external influence. The listing below gives the most appropriate indications for the five external flowers:

Star of Bethlehem

- ∾ Injuries
- ∾ Contusions
- ∾ Burns
- ∾ Sunburns
- ∾ Sun allergies
- ∾ Chemical burns

Gorse

- ∾ Local disturbances and results of injuries that have been unsuccessfully treated over a long time period

---

*The "external" or "outer" flowers (see *New Bach Flower Therapies*) combine the negative emotions, which deal with the emotions that result from reactions to external influences—for example, consequences of emotional shock, feeling overwhelmed by great challenges, and insecurity in a new stage of life. The external flowers are Aspen, Elm, Gorse, Star of Bethlehem, and Walnut.

ॐ Wounds or sores that do not heal

Elm

ॐ Muscle and joint pain after overexertion
ॐ Tennis elbow
ॐ Back and shoulder pain after heavy lifting
ॐ Muscle ache

Since these indications most often are associated with a lot of pain, an application of compresses is recommended. Elm is the flower for overexertion of any kind. If the overexertion has caused injury, combination with Star of Bethlehem is appropriate.

Walnut

ॐ Lacerations
ॐ Open wounds
ॐ Prevention against poor wound healing or excessive scar formation
ॐ Treatment of scars

Since the flowers should not be applied directly to the wound, internal use is generally recommended in the form of a water solution (two drops from the stock bottle in one 8 ounce glass of water). In acute cases, take one sip every fifteen to thirty minutes; otherwise sip 4 or 5 times through the day. In cases of acute injury a combination with Star of Bethlehem is appropriate.

Aspen

ॐ Results of ethereal influences

This indication needs to be based on a sensitive diagnosis. Inexplicable fears that occur in conjunction with physical symptoms can indicate Aspen.

THE TREATMENT OF SCARS

Under certain circumstances scars, even if they are small, can cause a variety of health disturbances. If the healing of a wound is incomplete, the scar will block energy flow at that location and a so-called disturbance field will develop, which can then trigger other disturbances at any place in the body. Keeping in mind that energy flows in the meridians correspond to measurable changes in skin resistance and that dysfunctional scars show a different skin resistance than their surrounding tissues, this concept of a disturbance field is quite reasonable.

It is rare that one can actually see from the outside that a scar represents a disturbance field; however, the aurically sensitive person can find a small indentation of the aura above the disturbed area. Otherwise, adequate information can only be gotten by measuring skin resistance or by administering a test treatment. Naturopathic doctors usually inject a local anesthetic below the scar. If the supposition was correct, all the symptoms caused by the scar will disappear within seconds.

Rubbing Walnut into the skin zone occupied by such a scar will have the same result as the injection. The application of the Bach Flower to the skin zone causes no pain. As well, it offers an advantage for scars around the mouth area, in such cases as tooth extraction or tonsil scars. To achieve the same effect as the injection, Walnut should be used undiluted; a few drops of the flower are applied on a cotton swab and brushed onto the scar. To assure complete healing for new scars, treatment with Walnut cream is also possible.

"SOUL COSMETIC"

Emotions that reveal themselves in the energy field can also, under certain circumstances, show up in the physical body. In such cases the skin becomes a mirror of our emotions—excitement becomes visible through blushing, shock reveals itself by paleness, insecurity causes increased sweating.

When we do not stay associated in our bodies at the time of emotial charge or when we carry an emotion inside us for a long period of time, the actual emotion will reflect itself as a disturbance in the skin's functions. For example, the feeling of being unclean will lead to skin disorders; if we separate ourselves from our surroundings, our skin will peel and a scaly "shield" will develop. Thus it is that our secret feelings, small and big, are made visible to the world. Our skin reveals things that we take great care to hide.

What makes more sense, then, than to treat negative emotions in the place where they become most visible—that is, in the face? Edward Bach used his flowers for cosmetic purposes. Nora Weeks writes:

A forty-year-old man had an ugly wart on his forehead, which influenced his well-being a great deal. He was a jovial type and felt most comfortable around his circle of friends, with whom he could talk about any conceivable topic, including his physical well-being. This kind of emotionally grounded state made it seem useful to prescribe Heather. Bach prescribed this remedy to him in the form of a lotion. Three weeks after the beginning of the treatment the wart was completely gone, without leaving a trace of a scar behind.[9]

Jens Eric Peterson also tells about a cosmetic treatment with Bach Flowers:

Girl, twelve years old. The girl had many pimples on her face. Despite the fact that her family doctor assured the mother that they would disappear by themselves over time, the girl felt very unhappy and did not have faith in herself anymore. She was a quiet, withdrawn child, who was always submerged in her daydreams. For her general state and her tendency of daydreaming Clematis was prescribed. The girl reacted quickly to this. She became much more alive and regained her interest in school and home. According to her mother, she even developed a great enthusiasm for many activities. Even her pimples vanished completely after the second small bottle of the flowers was used up.[10]

As these examples show, it is possible through the use of the type remedy to obtain positive results at any point of the body independent of the topography of the skin zones. As the type remedy is usually not able to be determined at the beginning of therapy, it is possible to combine some of the flowers into a cream, to use on a trial basis.

In selecting the proper flowers, the language of the organs usually offers important hints about the emotional ground state that has led to the main problem. Extremely sensitive skin, for example, indicates a quite vulnerable personality of the Star of Bethlehem type. Through the interview process, and in consideration of the patient's organ language, one can find those flowers that most closely relate to the disturbance of the skin. Those flowers can be used both as an internal application and as a cream. (The Bach Flowers can be added to commercially prepared and to homemade cosmetic creams.) When working with the flowers for cosmetic purposes, it is possible here to combine more than three flowers for a treatment.

Another possibility for the recognition of the underlying negative mental states that show up as skin problems is offered through the topography of skin zones. For example, wrinkles above the upper lip show a Willow state projected onto the skin. When strong feelings of dislike have triggered this state, the wrinkles will extend farther down below the corner of the mouth into the Holly zone, where they will occur as deep folds. The actual negative emotions might have already vanished, but the traces that the feeling inflicted into the skin continue to be visible.

Application Examples

For the treatment of acne in adolescence, the following flowers should be considered:

- ∾ Walnut for the transition into a new life phase;
- ∾ Crab Apple against the (mostly unconscious) fear of aroused sexuality and the feeling that it is something "dirty";
- ∾ Clematis for the state of dwelling in fantasies, typical for this stage in life.

In general, the use of collagen cream is not recommended for fighting acne, since it plugs the pores and thereby prevents detoxification of the skin. Noticeably pale skin can sometimes be an indication of a Clematis state, a state in which the person does not actively participate in life. Flabby skin points toward a listless disposition. The following flowers can be helpful in this case:

- ∾ Hornbeam for lack of enthusiasm or drive, in conjunction with fatigue and exhaustion due to continuous mental demand;
- ∾ Centaury for people who lack willpower, who cannot say no and consequently have been absolutely drained by other people;
- ∾ Wild Rose for people whose inner resignation has made them apathetic and indifferent. (Under certain circumstances, the Wild Rose state could have existed many years previously);
- ∾ Larch when there is no trust in one's own abilities;
- ∾ Mustard for people who suffer depressive phases, in which one's life appears to be senseless and empty.

Finally, it is important to state that the use of Bach Flowers for cosmetic purposes does not only serve the looks. As most of the treated skin areas are indeed disturbed zones, application to the skin will also help to unfold one's personality. For this reason, the phrase "soul cosmetic" seems to be appropriate indeed.

5
CASE HISTORIES

A young woman experienced much pain during her menstrual period. Since the Mimulus zone on the left side (see page 146) and the Olive zone on the right (see page 164) corresponded to the places where she felt pain during menstruation, she mixed a few drops of these two flowers into a salve base and rubbed it into the painful areas two to three times a day. After the first treatment the pain in her lower abdomen subsided. Three days later she had the sensation of an energy flow from head to toe. That sensation arose with every successive treatment, minimizing her chronic menstrual cramps.

> A fifty-four-year-old female patient suffered chronic, strong pains in her chest, which according to the medical diagnosis was a result of herpes zoster. Although confined to a small area, the pain was unbearable. Other treatment methods (neural therapy and ozone therapy) had been tried previously; even cortisone injections offered only short-term ease.
>
> After rubbing Honeysuckle onto the corresponding skin zone, the pains instantly dissipated. After a few hours they slowly reappeared, and the patient applied the Honeysuckle again. She followed this course of treatment for several days. After five days not only had her chest pain completely vanished, but the depression she had had for many years was also gone. This depression was always connected with a feeling of yearning (a Honeysuckle characteristic), which she was unable to define previously.

The same patient came back some time later complaining of a terrible headache. She had already tried several pain medications, which did not work at all. I injected a homeopathic medication into some points indicated

28

by a Kirlian photograph. After the injections the patient was pain free. She was advised to rub Rock Water onto the affected area if the pains came back. A week later she told me that the success of the initial treatment lasted for only one day. The pain returned full force the next day, but after an application of Rock Water, it completely disappeared.

> A thirty-four-year-old female patient came to the office with shoulder and neck pain that had grown worse over time. A month-long pain therapy had not only been unsuccessful, but her pain had increased to the point where she had to take medication to make it through the day.

When she came to see me, the woman had already missed several days of work due to the intensity of the pain. I rubbed two drops of Oak onto the painful areas around the neck and shoulder region. Afterward she reported that her pain had initially disappeared, but then moved to the front and was even stronger. She especially felt a lot of pain on the left side, in the area around the thyroid gland and the sternocleidomastoid muscle. Vervain flower dominates this area.

I trickled three drops of Vervain onto the painful area, whereby the patient fell into a state of trance. After the application of the drops she entered a state of peaceful relaxation, then fell asleep on the chair. Later she told me that she was aware of everything around her, while her body had fallen into a warm, resting state.

When she came back to my office three days later, she told me that she had not gotten any sleep in the days before the treatment. She sensed that when the flowers were rubbed in, the body had become aware on an ethereal level of the ideal equilibrium between the active principle (yang) and the passive principle (yin). Since she had exploited her health during the days before the treatment, she realized that the balance between activity and rest had been massively disturbed. As a result, the body had initiated necessary steps to force her to rest, in order to restore her physical balance. That was why she had fallen asleep immediately after the treatment.

For preventive purposes, I suggested that she do further applications to the zones in the form of compresses; however, the pain did not recur.

> A thirty-six-year-old man came to my office for help with a fistula in the region around the anus. He complained of difficulties with sitting because the spot was so painful.

I applied two drops of Sweet Chestnut to the zone around the area, and the pain lessened in minutes. After five minutes the pain was completely gone and the patient was able to sit down without discomfort.

The fistula healed slowly with home treatments (compresses). After four weeks, the fistula was hardly visible.

> A forty-seven-year-old woman consulted me regarding pain in her sinuses that radiated into her ears. Her doctor found a cyst in her left sinus cavity, which he wanted to remove surgically.

After application of the Oak remedy to the left cheek and the area behind the left ear, she told me that she could sense a rushing that extended from the ear toward her sinuses—she characterized it as a feeling of forced air being blown through to free her ducts and cavities. Eight weeks later, after further treatment with compresses on the area, a follow-up visit was scheduled with her physician. The result was quite remarkable: There was no more talk about surgery.

> A forty-six-year-old woman complained that her menses had not come for a long time. Her doctor attributed this to menopause and told her not to worry about it. I am of the opinion that a woman's menstrual cycle should be encouraged to last as far into her midlife as possible. This cycle represents an energetic charge and discharge that finds its release through the monthly bleeding. A physical cleansing simultaneously takes place.

With these thoughts in mind, one should always ask what triggered the hormonal disturbance, when the problem is in connection with the menses. In many cases such a problem is based on emotional causes; in this case, the patient was not at ease with her own sexuality. She experienced feelings of guilt when she had sex with her husband.

After application of a few drops of the Pine remedy to the zone around the sacrum, she felt as though fire was streaming through her lower abdomen. This state suddenly appeared and then disappeared just as quickly. A sensation of heat remained, however, and persisted for quite a while longer. The woman received advice to apply compresses of the Pine flower to this zone daily. After three weeks she came back to the office radiant with joy and told me that her period had returned.

> A seventy-four-year-old woman came to my office because of periodic bronchitis. Her physician had helped her initially, but the pain and the cough recurred again and again. She indicated a point on her chest where she experienced extreme pain even at the slightest touch.

After Oak was applied to the zone, she had the feeling that her rib cage had become lighter. After approximately one minute, her pain was completely gone. I explained to her how to correctly use the compresses so that she could continue treatments at home. Two weeks later she came back to my office and reported that she had no further coughing spells following the treatment.

A thirty-three-year-old woman came to my office due to an enlarged thyroid gland. She could not stand hot weather—it made the sensation of pressure in her thyroid gland unbearable, and she would suffer with difficulties swallowing and breathing and would get very lightheaded. She had been treated unsuccessfully with medications for one year.

After a rubdown of the thyroid zone with the Bach Flower Vervain, the patient had the feeling that her thyroid gland was steadily growing and would soon burst. The pressure relocated to the center of the gland, and I applied Water Violet to that spot. A short time later she had the sensation of pressure flowing downward, then completely disappearing. She was instructed to rub herself down daily with these flowers.

Weeks later the woman reported that she was symptom free and had never tolerated hot weather so well.

A seventy-six-year-old man consulted me because of constant asthma attacks. His breathing was heavy and wheezy. The strongest allopathic medicines were unable to help him. His chest was full of pain and at night he was most uncomfortable, which made him wake up early in the morning completely exhausted.

Oak was rubbed into a spot on his chest and Mimulus was applied to a zone on his back. He reported a sudden stinging sensation in his chest, and his spine felt hot in the upper region. After five minutes, his chest felt freer than it had felt for quite a long time. He was instructed to apply both flowers at home, in the form of compresses.

When he returned to my office one week later, the success of the treatment still persisted. He was surprised that the drops had had such a powerful effect on his lungs, especially given that the drops had been applied externally only. He chose not to schedule an additional appointment, fearing that his symptoms might reappear if he were treated again.

A forty-four-year-old woman had an acute cold with a running nose, cough, and bronchial complaints. Her breathing had become extremely difficult. Listening to her chest, I heard loud crackling noises. After a few drops of Centaury were applied, her breathing became easier and the rasping noises could no longer be heard.

A twenty-two-year-old man with an impatient disposition suffered with hair loss and pain in his scalp. His hair was already thin, and he was afraid he would be bald soon. The episodic bouts of pain were accompanied by much hair loss. His scalp was very sensitive to the touch. The complaints had started in the Impatiens zone and spread throughout the head.

The patient received a hair tonic consisting of distilled water, to which some drops of Impatiens were added. In addition I gave him a mineral mixture to exclude a possible deficiency as the cause, and a flower mixture for internal use. The flower mixture changed during the course of the treatment.

After three weeks the patient was almost pain free. There was no more hair loss and the scalp pains reappeared only occasionally—mostly during phases of impatience—and vanished within minutes after application of the hair tonic.

A thirty-one-year-old patient arrived with an acute headache and tension in his neck and shoulders. He had awakened in that state that morning. After rubbing Olive into his shoulders and Water Violet on his neck, he immediately became symptom free.

An older patient complained about heart pain. He experienced an unpleasant sensation of pressure in the area around the heart which got worse if he was in a conversation over a long period of time. He reported feeling as though his heart was contracting and his pulse could stumble; he sometimes expected that his heart would stop beating at any minute. A round of clinical tests had shown no disturbances.

The patient received a Centaury cream, with instructions to apply it twice a day to the area around the heart. On the third day he reported that he was almost symptom free, as if somebody had flipped a switch. A week after treatment began, his complaints were gone.

A five-year-old boy suffered from a stomach ache. Since the pain was localized in the Rock Rose zone, he was asked if recently he had been terribly afraid, maybe even scared to death (a characteristic of Rock Rose). As a result he talked about an event that happened several weeks previously.

After a single rubdown with Rock Rose, the boy was completely pain free.

A young man complained of a dull pressure in his forehead and a feeling of drowsiness. He had not been sleeping much.

After a few drops of Olive were rubbed on his forehead, he immediately had a feeling of everything around him becoming much brighter and clearer. The feeling of drowsiness dissolved within seconds.

A thirty-year-old patient complained about a headache. Examination of her aura showed that the Larch zone around the umbilicus appeared to be especially disturbed. After Larch was applied, her headache disappeared. Since she had suffered a lack of self-esteem ever since she was a child (a Larch characteristic), she continued the treatment at home.

In the days that followed, she experienced an emotional lift. Later she told me that she had a not experienced feelings of low self-esteem after the first treatment. Instead she experienced an indescribably high feeling that enabled her to do things she thought she was unable to do.

A thirty-year-old patient complained of pain and tension around the seventh cervical vertebra. After Wild Rose was rubbed onto it, the pain immediately subsided and the muscles started to relax. Her complaints did not recur.

A sixty-year-old woman was experiencing difficulty with her breathing. Time and again she had a cold feeling in her lungs, as if she was breathing cold air. It was difficult for her to take a deep breath.

A single rubbing of the neck with Vervain was enough to eliminate the problem once and for all. A few seconds following the treatment she was able to breathe normally again.

A friend told me of a pressure sensation in her right forehead and her sense of decreased vision in her right eye. It felt as if an eye shield was hindering her vision. According to my advice, she rubbed the area with Olive. The pressure in her forehead immediately dissolved, the feeling in the eye disappeared, and her vision returned to normal.

A fifty-nine-year-old patient had pain in his buttocks. He had been treated homeopathically for numerous other complaints, and all of them had improved after treatment with a high-potency homeopathic remedy; however, the pain in his buttocks remained resistant to therapy.

The patient was advised to use compresses of Sweet Chestnut daily. Four weeks later he reported that all his complaints were completely gone.

During his life this patient had often experienced states of extreme desperation. Although the events that brought on such states happened a long time ago—the first one when he was one year old—the emotions remained stored in his body.

> A thirty-two-year-old female had suffered for a year with a strange tingling in a localized spot at the left side of her head. She also occasionally experienced a burn or a twinge which extended into her neck. She had been clinically examined with all the latest modalities, but a cause for the tingling could not be determined. Even the CAT scan did not offer a conclusion.

This woman simultaneously suffered strong fears. She constantly had the feeling that somebody was on her back and urging her to do something. The feeling was especially severe when she drove her car. She always thought somebody was driving with her and was pushing her foot against the gas pedal, which she then had to retract with all her might. These events made her feel nauseated. Her circulation decreased and she felt as though she would collapse.

Often she felt drunk and walked alongside a wall for support. Often she would panic as she crossed the street. She was constantly afraid that something might happen to her or that she would fall over. She was afraid of going crazy.

After an application of Vine to the affected area, the tingling turned into a throbbing pain, which shortly thereafter radiated into her neck. After rubbing Water Violet on her neck the pressure and the heavy feeling eased immediately, but she felt a pain in her left shoulder that radiated into her arm. After an application of Gorse she was momentarily free of symptoms.

After half an hour the tingling started up again. I dropped two drops of Aspen onto her tongue and rubbed Willow onto her lower spine. Immediately, the tingling stopped. She received instructions to apply Vine, Water Violet, and Gorse daily to the respective areas in undiluted form. The oral mixture contained Aspen, Cherry Plum, and Willow. Star of Bethlehem was added due to emotional trauma in her past. The decompensation flowers Pine, Beech, and Mustard found through the interview were also added.

Due to the external flowers the total number of flowers exceeded the standard maximum of seven. In this case it was unavoidable since on the one hand, one has to give the flowers belonging to the reacting skin zones, and on the other hand, one has to pay attention to the states of decompensation, which were very strongly formed and needed to be addressed first. An

34

overreaction can be avoided by not giving the external mixture simultaneously with the internal one. The later one should not contain more than seven flowers. In further mixtures the number of flowers used was gradually reduced.

After three months I saw the patient again. She felt much better overall. The tingling was almost gone. It rarely resurfaced and always immediately disappeared again after a treatment. The sensation of somebody driving her from behind was completely gone.

> A twenty-six-year-old patient complained of always feeling tired. After Wild Rose was rubbed on the appropriate zone on her right arm, she at once had the feeling of becoming more awake.

A therapy-resistant state of deep fatigue is quite common and sometimes can be attributed to a past state of resignation. Most often it will vanish quickly after treatment of this particular zone. Quite frequently we were able to observe that a rubbing of this area works just like a cup of coffee: Often, the feeling of being more awake occurred as soon as the drops had been applied to the skin. For the Wild Rose zone one should not apply the flower remedy directly from the stock bottle.

> A fifty-six-year-old patient complained about much tension in the shoulder and neck area. She could turn her head without strain only to her left side. When she tried to move her head in the other direction, the tension in her neck muscles prevented rotation.

After the zone around the seventh cervical vertebra was rubbed with Wild Rose, the tension eased and she was able to move her head freely again.

6
FURTHER THERAPEUTIC POSSIBILITIES

In addition to the treatment possibilities described in this book and in *New Bach Flower Therapies,* there are further forms of treatment based mainly on the concept of the tracks. The relationship of the tracks to each other offers valuable diagnostic information as well as new treatment opportunities. The effect of the flowers can be intensified through this method of treatment, which can be very significant in therapy-resistant cases.

During our practical work we discovered points on the body that, when tested for their sensitivity to pressure, made it possible to draw diagnostic conclusions about the track. These points are part of a whole system of points which have a direct relationship to the Bach flowers. They offer a possibility for the therapist to continue the work with the flowers on the skin even when the illness has already progressed far into the viscera, and the potential of the flowers is no longer sufficient to eliminate the complaints. Instead of using other treatment methods in these cases, it is possible with the help of these points to transfer the Bach Flower diagnostic directly into body therapy and to treat the points that correspond to the particular flowers. Depending on the severity of the illness the points are injected with homeopathic remedies or radiated with colors. In many cases acupressure is also sufficient.

The treatment of the flower points in most cases will bring instant relief of pain in the area associated with the flowers. Sometimes physical reactions in other skin zones also associated with the flower will occur immediately after the treatment. We observed a temporary flare-up of the emotional symptoms associated with the flowers of the treated points, not unlike the healing crises that occur with homeopathy. It is our feeling that these reactions offer proof of the existence of the tracks.

There are other treatment possibilities with Bach Flowers and the newly derived diagnostic and therapy methods under trial. The underlying goal of this research is the creation of a holistic therapy concept in which Bach Flower Therapy is central to the therapy for physical illnesses and does not serve only as a supportive therapy for emotional balancing.

7

Topographic Atlas of the Skin Zones

Finding the Zones on the Back

∾

Finding the skin zones on the back can be made easier by marking the palpable spinal areas with a marker or a cosmetic eyeliner. To locate the individual vertebrae it is easiest to identify a prominent point and count either up or down from there. One such point is the seventh cervical vertebra at the base of the neck. When bending the head forward, it will show in the uppermost region of the shoulders as the most prominent vertebra. Below the seventh cervical vertebra are the twelve thoracic vertebrae and the five lumbar vertebrae. The other easy-to-locate point along the spine is the fourth lumbar vertebra, located horizontal to the upper edge of the iliac crest. This vertebra is best found by placing the hands on the uppermost points of the hips and drawing a line from each point to the spine. The two lines will connect at the fourth lumbar vertebra.

AGRIMONY

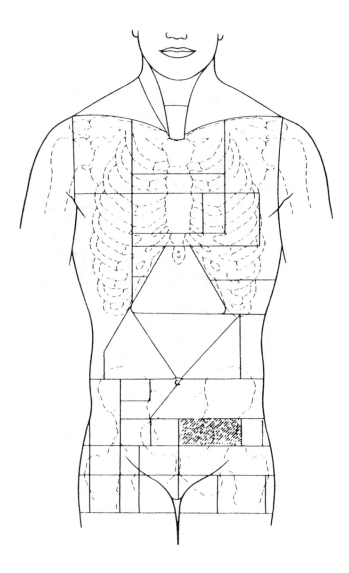

The Agrimony zone on the left side begins halfway between the upper pubic edge and the navel and ends at the level of the pubic hair line. The inner border is the midline of the body. The zone extends 6 finger widths horizontally from the midline.

AGRIMONY

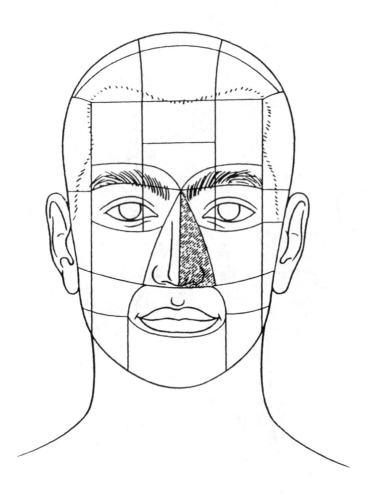

The Agrimony zone on the left half of the nose extends from the midpoint of the eyebrows straight down the center of the nose to its tip and around its base.

AGRIMONY

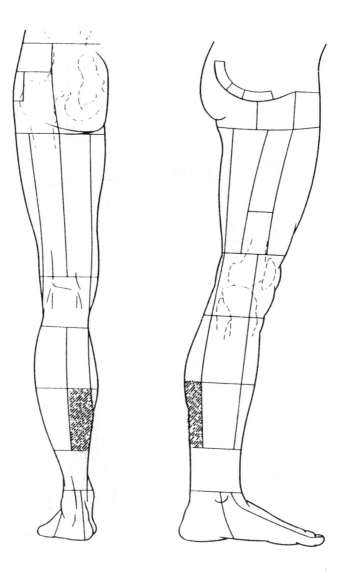

The Agrimony zone located on the left lower leg begins 4 finger widths from the upper edge of the left inner ankle bone and extends upward 6 finger widths. The back border is located in the middle of the calf on a line extending from the Achilles tendon to the back of the knee. The zone extends 3 finger widths forward toward the inside of the leg.

AGRIMONY

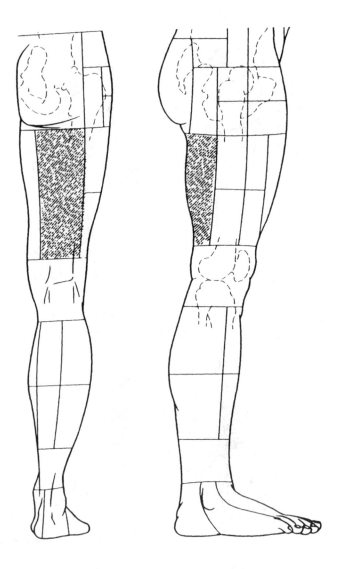

The Agrimony flower also covers a zone at the back of the upper right thigh. It begins 1 finger width below the fold of the buttock and ends 1 finger width above the kneecap. The side borders are located 2½ finger widths from the middle of the knee on both sides.

ASPEN

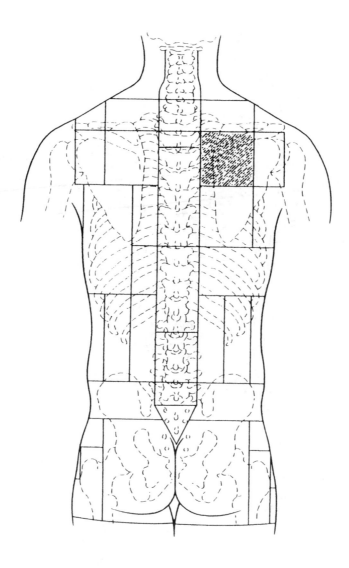

The Aspen zone on the back originates at the level of the second thoracic vertebra and ends at the level of the fifth thoracic vertebra. The inner border is located 2 finger widths to the right of the transverse processes and extends 6 finger widths to the right of that.

ASPEN

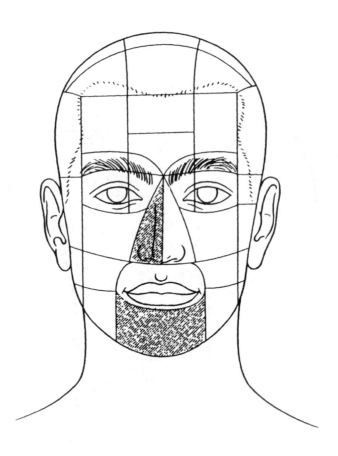

On the face, the Aspen flower covers the right half of the nose. The zone extends from the midpoint of the eyebrows straight down to the tip of the nose and around its base. The zone also stretches from the bottom edge of the lower lip to the edge of the chin. The outer margins run from the sides of the mouth to the rim of the chin.

ASPEN

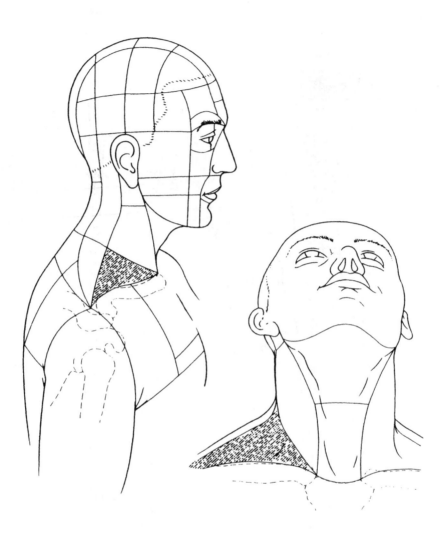

The Aspen zone continues on the right side from the side margin of the tra-pezius muscle along the upper edge of the collarbone. The intersection of two lines extending upward from the front and rear shoulder folds would mark the outer border of this skin zone. The inner border is located at the base of the neck. This zone is often painful on palpation.

ASPEN

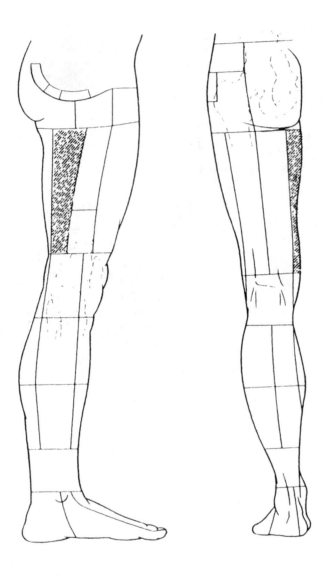

The Aspen zone also lies on the left inner thigh. It begins 1 finger width below the fold of the buttock and ends 1 finger width above the kneecap. The upper front margin is located 1 finger width to the left of the body's midline. The lower frontal margin is 4 finger widths to the side of the kneecap. The zone extends $2\frac{1}{2}$ finger widths to the left of the front margin.

BEECH

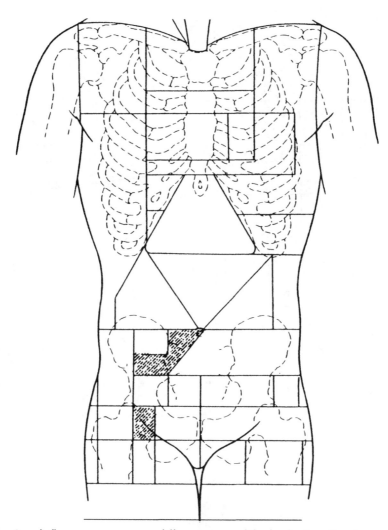

The Beech flower covers many different areas of the body. Two Beech zones are located on the right side of the abdomen. The upper zone begins at the navel and extends approximately 3 finger widths horizontally. The inner and bottom margins begin 5 finger widths below this point, extending approximately 3 finger widths to the right outer margin and sloping diagonally upward to the navel. The outer margin abuts the nipple line.

The lower abdominal zone extends from the hip socket to the level of the groin. The inner edge lies 4 finger widths to the right of the midline; the zone extends 2 finger widths to the right.

BEECH

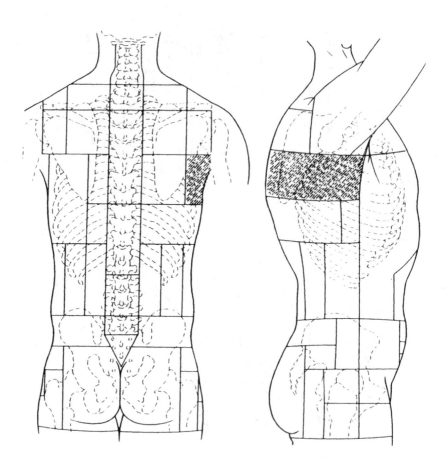

Another Beech zone originates on the back at the level of the fifth thoracic vertebra and ends at the level of the eighth thoracic vertebra. The inner border is located 8 finger widths to the right of the midline. The outer border is formed by an imaginary vertical extension of the front axial fold.

BEECH

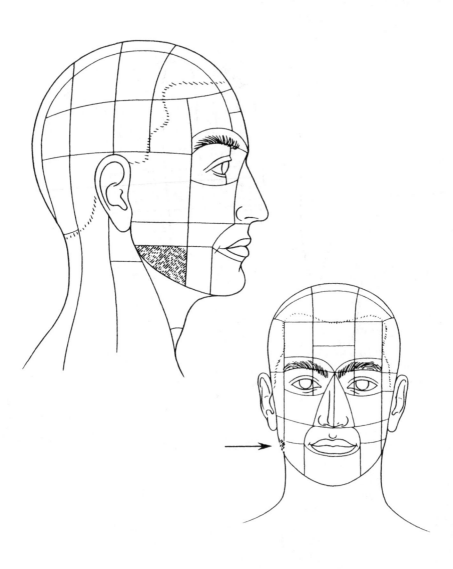

The facial zone for the Beech flower begins at a line horizontal to the right corner of the mouth and follows the lower margin of the jaw. The front border is formed by a vertical line through the outer corner of the eyebrow, the back border by the jawbone.

BEECH

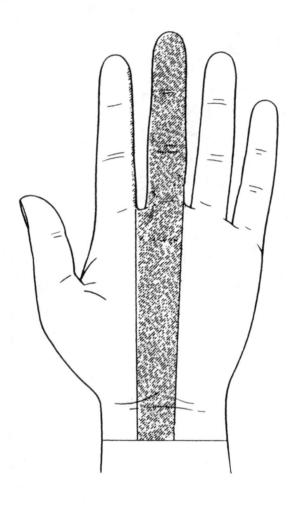

Another Beech zone lies on the inside of the left hand. It extends from a point 1 finger width above the wrist to the tip of the index and middlefingers. The left border begins 1 finger width inside the left outer edge of the wrist and runs to the right edge of the index finger. The right border starts at the middle of the wrist and runs to the right corner of the middle finger. The zones of the palm side of the hand extend to the midline side of the fingers.

BEECH

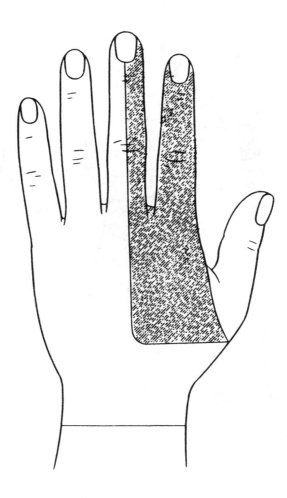

The Beech flower also applies to a zone on the back of the left hand that extends 2 finger widths above the wrist to the tips of the index and middle fingers. The zone runs from the inner corner of the index fingernail along its edge to the base of the thumb. The outside border is located on a vertical line running through the middle of the index finger.

BEECH

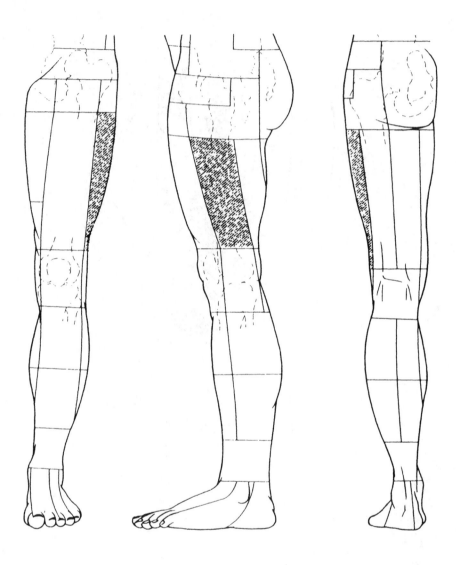

Another Beech zone is located on the outside of the left thigh, beginning 1 finger width below the fold of the buttock. The side margins abut the vertical lines of the front and rear axial folds; the lower margin lies 1 finger width above the kneecap. The front border is 2 finger widths to the side of the kneecap; the back border is 4 finger widths behind the kneecap.

Beech

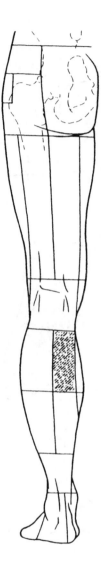

The Beech flower also applies to the back of the left calf. It begins 3½ finger widths below the left kneecap and extends 6 finger widths downward. The outside margin lies in the middle of the calf on an imaginary line stretching from the Achilles tendon to the middle of the knee. The inside margin lies 3 finger widths to the right.

BEECH

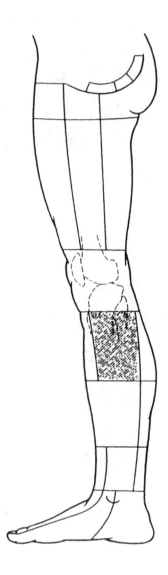

Another Beech zone found on the legs is located to the inside of the right knee. The zone begins 3½ finger widths below the right kneecap and extends 6 finger widths downward. The front border begins at the inside edge of the kneecap; the back border lies 5 finger widths away.

BEECH

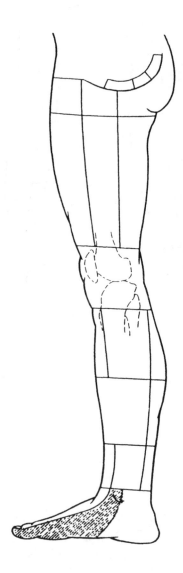

The Beech zone that covers the area on the right foot begins at the upper edge of the inner ankle bone and extends to the outer edge of the big toenail. The back border runs from the back of the ankle bone in a mild slope down to the arch of the foot.

BEECH

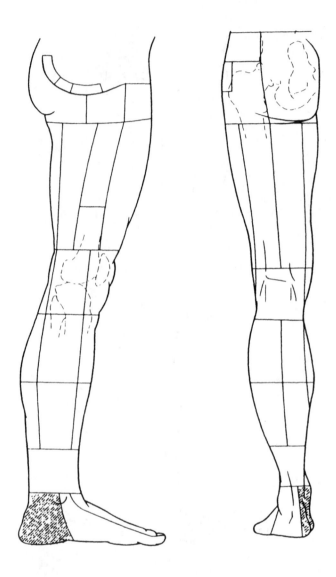

The last Beech zone originates on the left foot at the upper margin of the inner ankle bone and ends at the heel. The border in the back is formed by the Achilles tendon; the border in the front extends from the ankle bone in a mild slope to the back of the arch.

CENTAURY

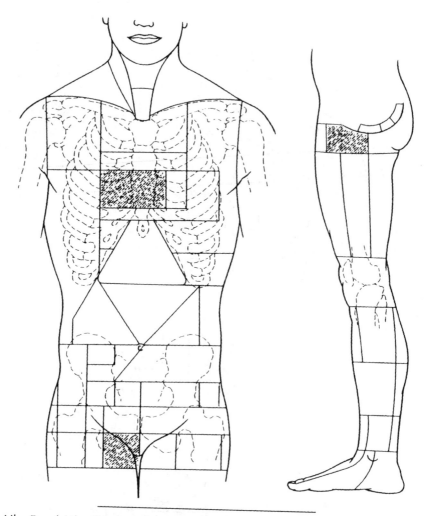

Like Beech, the Centaury flower also applies to several zones on the body. On the front of the body, the upper zone begins in the area of the third inter- costal and ends at the sixth intercostal. The left edge lies 2 finger widths to the left of the body's midline; the right edge ends 4 finger widths to the right of the midline.

The lower zone begins at the lower edge of the pubic bone and ends 1 finger width below an imaginary line from the buttock fold to the front. This zone encompasses the genitals. The inner border is formed by the body's midline; the zone extends 4 finger widths to the right.

CENTAURY

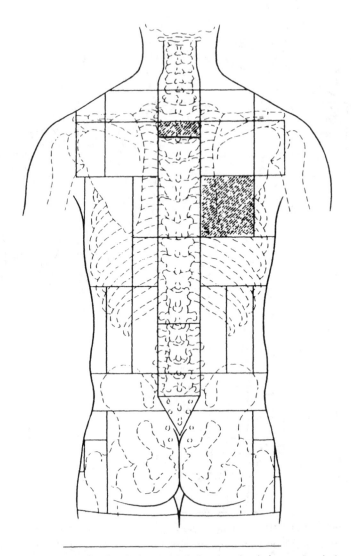

The upper zone on the back begins at the level of the second thoracic vertebra and extends to the third thoracic vertebra. The borders are 2 finger widths to the left and right of the spinal column.

The lower zone lies on the right side of the back, starting at the level of the fifth thoracic vertebra and ending at the level of the eighth thoracic vertebra. The inner border lies 2 finger widths to the right of the midline; its outer border lies 6 finger widths to the right.

CENTAURY

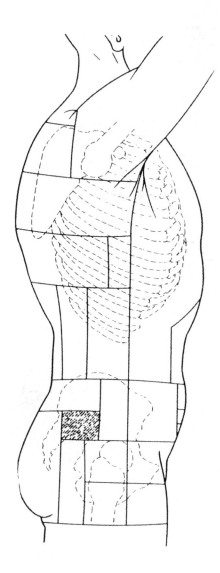

The Centaury zone on the right side of the body begins on a line extending downward from the iliac crest and ends at a point level with the top of the pubic bone. The zone extends 4½ finger widths toward the back.

CENTAURY

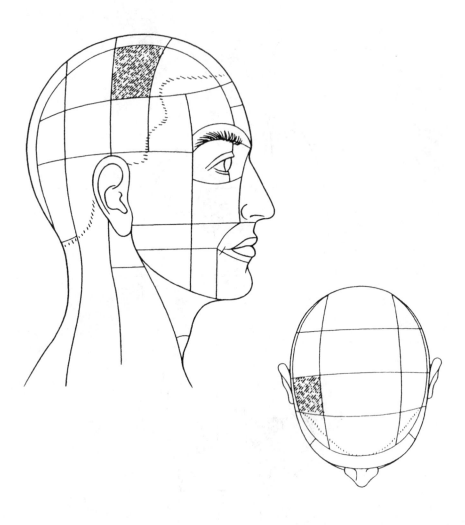

There are two Centaury zones on the head. One zone begins 1½ finger widths to the right of the head's midline and ends 3 finger widths above the tip of the right ear. The back border aligns vertically with the tip of the ear, with the zone extending 3 finger widths forward from there.

CENTAURY

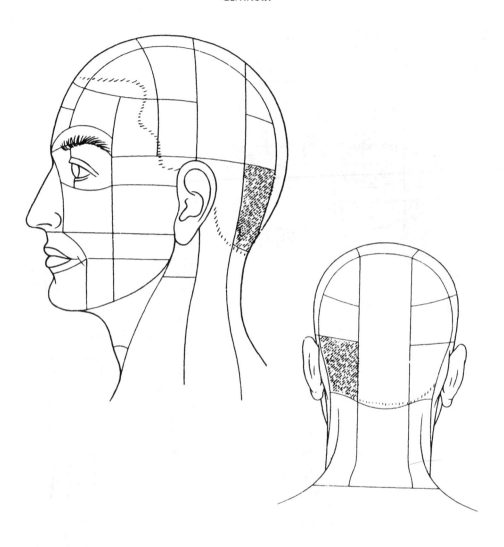

A second Centaury zone on the head begins at the left side on a horizontal line stretching from the top of the ear to the lower edge of the skull. The front border lies 2 finger widths behind the ear, the zone extending 3 finger widths toward the back.

CENTAURY

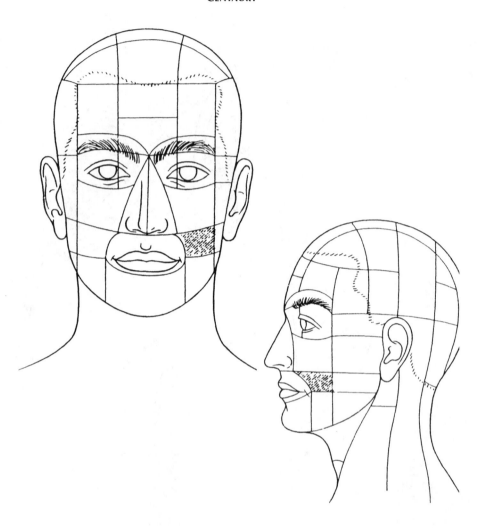

This Centaury zone is located on the left facial hemisphere. It begins on a horizontal line at the bottom of the nose and ends on a horizontal line at the corner of the mouth. The inner border lies on a curved line from the nose to the left corner of the mouth. The outer border is formed by a vertical line running through the left corner of the left eyebrow.

CENTAURY

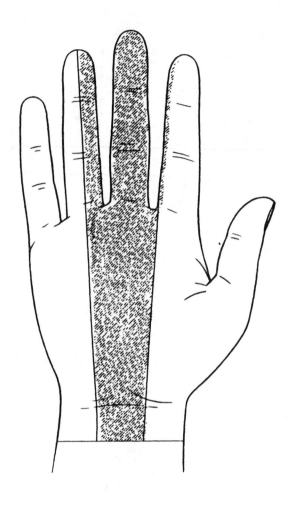

The Centaury zone located on the palm side of the right hand runs from 1 finger width above the wrist fold to the tips of the index, middle, and ring fingers. The right margin begins 1 finger width inside the lateral edge of the wrist, the zone extending upward to the left edge of the index finger. The left margin begins 1 finger width to the right of the wrist's medial edge, the zone extending upward to the middle of the ring finger. The zones of the palm side of the hand extend to the midline of the side of the fingers.

CENTAURY

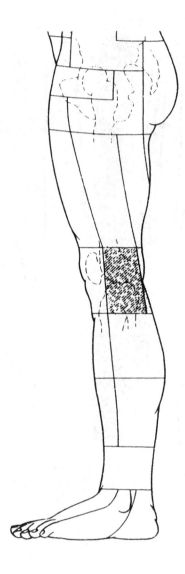

There are several Centaury zones on the leg and foot. One is located on the lateral side of the left knee. It begins 2 finger widths to the side of the left kneecap and extends 4 finger widths to the back. Its upper border is 1 finger width above the kneecap; its lower border is 3½ finger widths below the kneecap.

Centaury

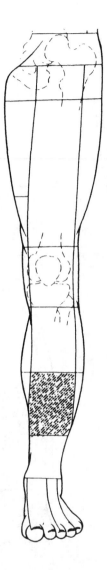

Another Centaury zone on the leg begins 4 finger widths above the upper edge of the inner ankle bone and extends upward 6 finger widths. The inner border is located on the inner edge of the shin, the outer border on a line that runs from 2 finger widths to the side of the kneecap to the outer tip of the ankle bone.

CENTAURY

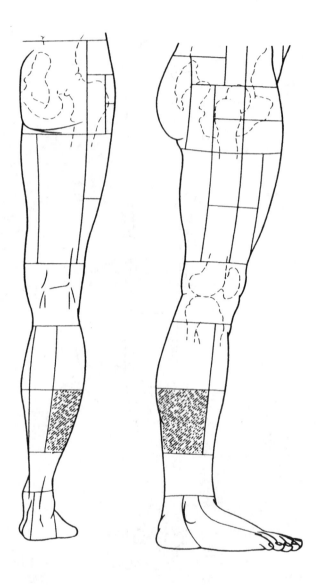

The Centaury zone on the right calf begins 4 finger widths above the upper edge of the ankle bone and extends four finger widths upward. The rear margin lies in the middle of the calf on an imaginary line from the Achilles tendon to the middle of the knee, the front margin on a vertical line 2 finger widths to the side of the kneecap.

CENTAURY

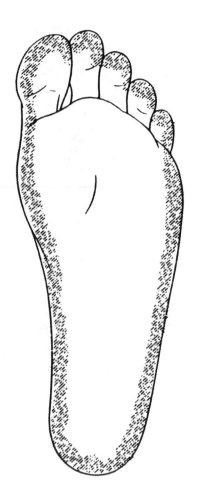

The Centaury zone covers the entire sole of the left foot including the plantar side of the toes.

CENTAURY

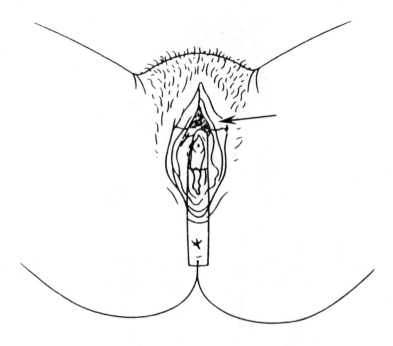

The Centaury flower zone also covers the clitoris, ending at its lower rim.

CERATO

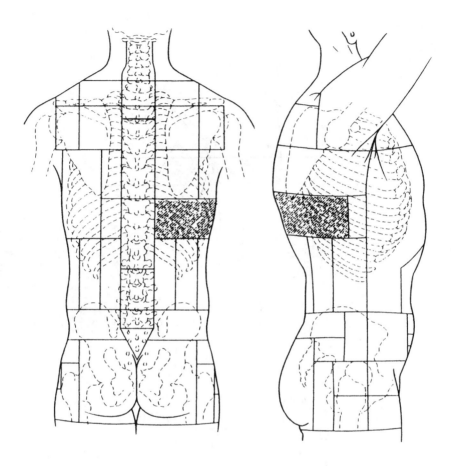

The Cerato zone on the back begins at the level of the eighth thoracic vertebra and ends at the level of the eleventh thoracic vertebra. The inside border lies 2 finger widths to the right of the midline of the back and extends laterally to align with the axial fold.

CERATO

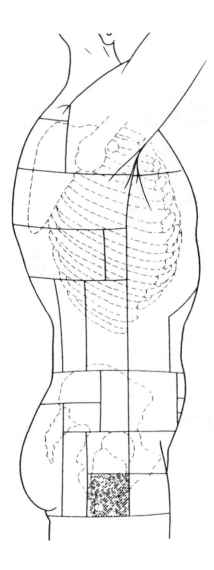

At the right hip, the Cerato zone begins horizontally 1 finger width below the tailbone, in an area bordered vertically by extensions of the front and back axial folds. The lower border of this zone aligns horizontally 1 finger width below the fold of the buttock.

CERATO

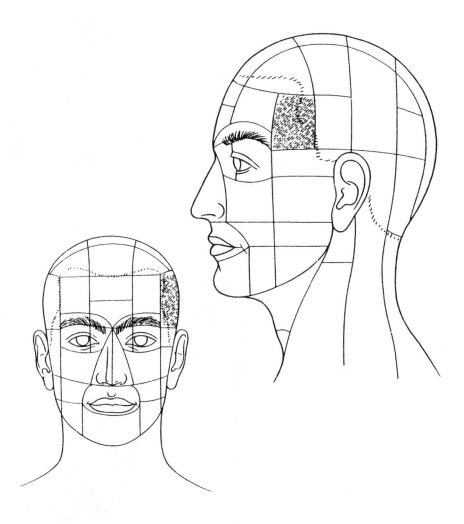

The Cerato zone located on the left side of the head begins at the level of the hairline and ends at the outer corner of the eyebrow. The zone extends 2½ finger widths to the back.

CERATO

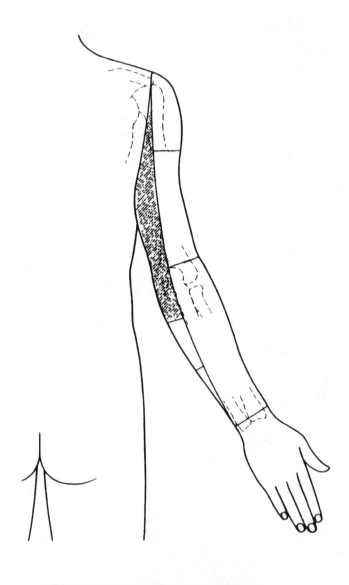

The Cerato zone on the right arm begins in the middle of the right axial fold and extends down the arm to 2 finger widths below the elbow. The inside border of the zone runs along the inside edge of the biceps muscle. The outside border is located on a vertical line 3 finger widths to the right of the axial fold with the arm extended. In the shoulder area the zone forms a triangle, the tip of the triangle lying just above the axial fold.

CERATO

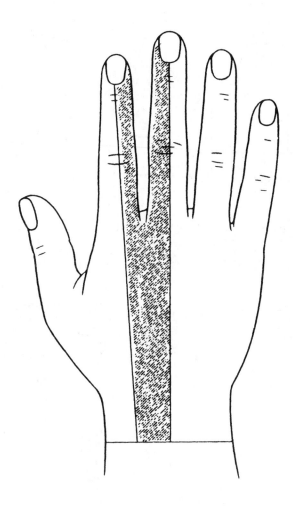

On the back of the right hand, the Cerato zone begins 1 finger width above the wrist fold and extends to the tips of the index and middle fingers. The right border runs from the middle of the wrist to the middle of the middle finger. The left border begins 1 finger width to the side of the wrist and runs to the middle of the index finger. The zones on the palm meet the zones at the back of the hand on the sides of the fingers.

CHERRY PLUM

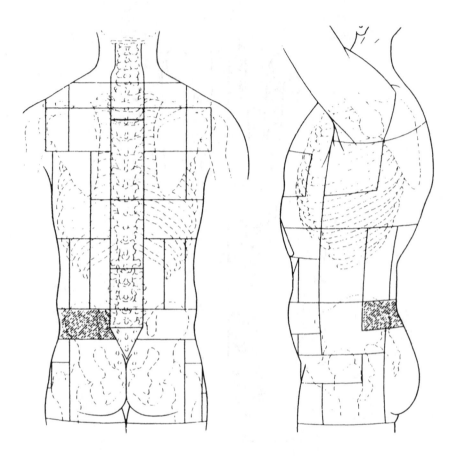

The Cherry Plum zone on the back begins at the level of the fourth lumbar vertebra and extends downward to the level of the sacral crest. The inside edge at the upper half of this zone lies 2 finger widths to the side of the midline. At the level of the sacral crest the border slopes toward the anal fold. The outer margin aligns vertically with the rear axial fold.

CHERRY PLUM

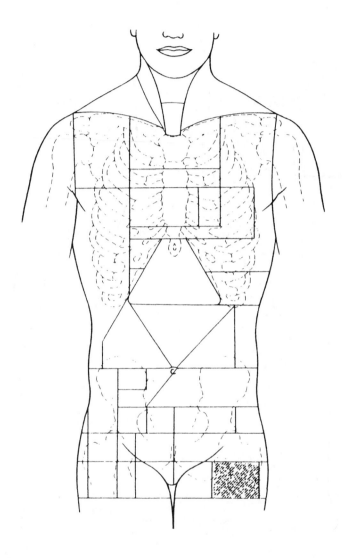

The Cherry Plum zone on the front of the body begins at the level of the pubis and ends 1 finger width below an imaginary line that would extend frontward from the fold of the buttock. The inner edge lies 4 finger widths to the side of the midline and extends laterally to align vertically with the front axial fold.

CHERRY PLUM

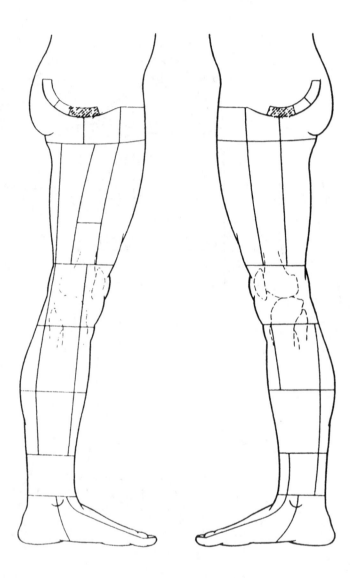

This Cherry Plum zone corresponds with the prostate gland. It extends from above the anus (where the red coloration of the anus ends) to the base of the scrotum. The side margins of the zone end in the groin fold.

CHERRY PLUM

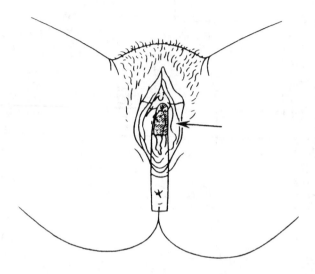

For women, the Cherry Plum zone corresponds with the so-called G-spot. The zone begins at the upper rim of the vagina and ends below the clitoris. It is bordered on the sides by the labia.

CHESTNUT BUD

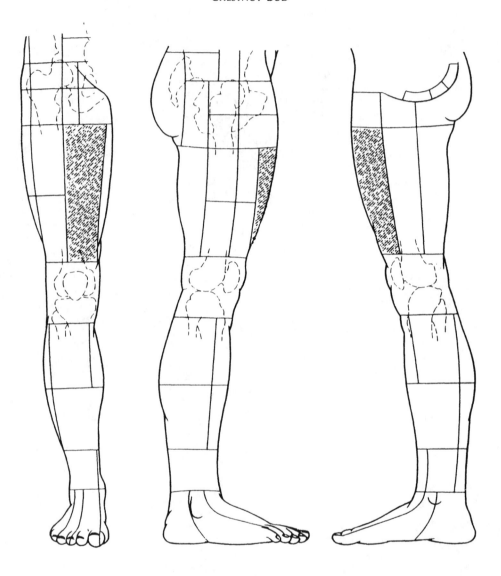

The two Chestnut Bud zones are located on the leg. The zone on the right thigh begins on a horizontal line extending 1 finger width below the fold of the buttock and ends 1 finger width above the kneecap. The outer border lies 1 finger width inside the outer edge of the kneecap. The lower end of the inner border lies 2 finger widths to the left of the kneecap; the upper end is 4 finger widths from the body's midline.

CHESTNUT BUD

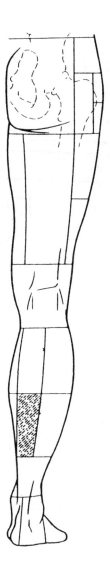

The Chestnut Bud zone on the right calf begins 4 finger widths above the upper margin of the inner ankle bone and ends 6 finger widths above that. The back border is located at the middle of the calf on a line that extends from the Achilles tendon to the middle of the knee. The zone extends 3 finger widths toward the front.

CHICORY

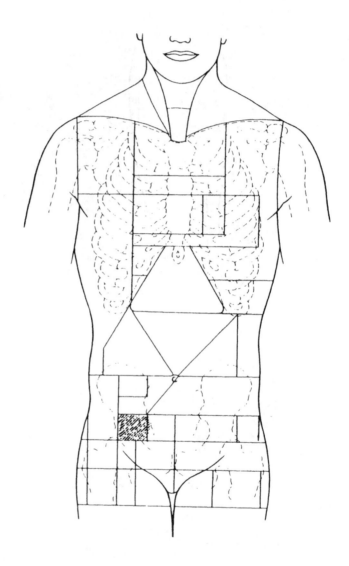

The Chicory zone on the trunk begins at the anterior superior iliac spine, halfway between the pubic bone and the navel. The zone extends downward to the pubic bone. The medial border begins 3 finger widths from the midline and extends laterally another 3 finger widths.

CHICORY

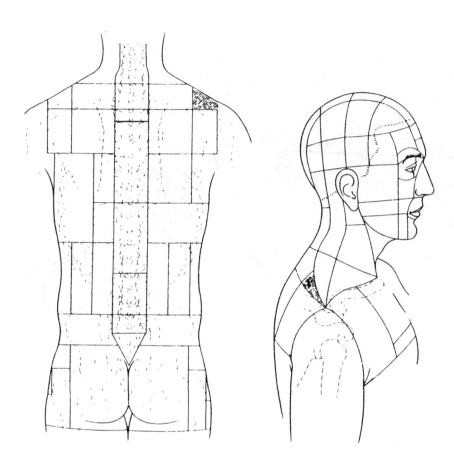

The Chicory zone on the right shoulder begins at the level of the sixth cervical vertebra at the shoulder margin of the trapezius muscle and ends at the level of the second thoracic vertebra. The border on the right aligns vertically with the axial fold; the zone extends 3 finger widths toward the midline.

CHICORY

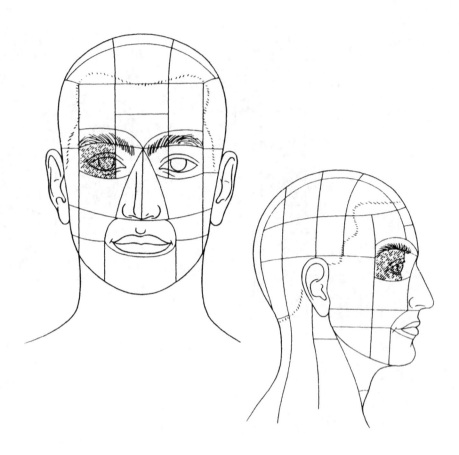

The Chicory zone at the right eye begins at the lower end of the eyebrow and ends at the lower edge of the eye socket. The inner border aligns with the inside edge of the iris; the outer border aligns with the outer edge of the eyebrow.

Chicory

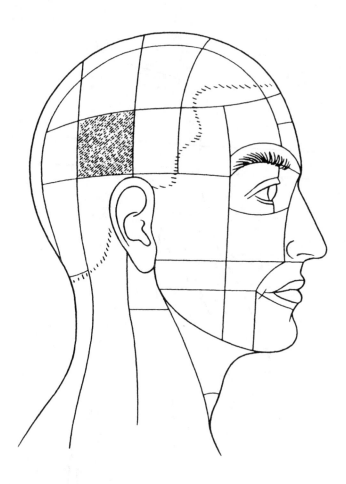

The Chicory zone on the right side of the head begins at the upper edge of the ear and extends 3 finger widths upward. The front border aligns vertically with the tip of the ear; the zone extends 3 finger widths backward.

CHICORY

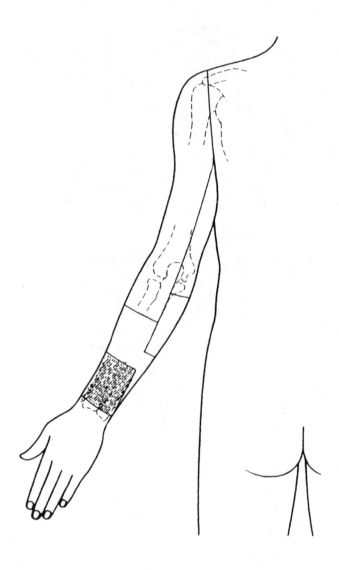

The Chicory zone on the left lower arm begins 1 finger width above the wrist and extends 5 finger widths upward. The side borders are formed by the lateral edges of the radius and the ulna.

CHICORY

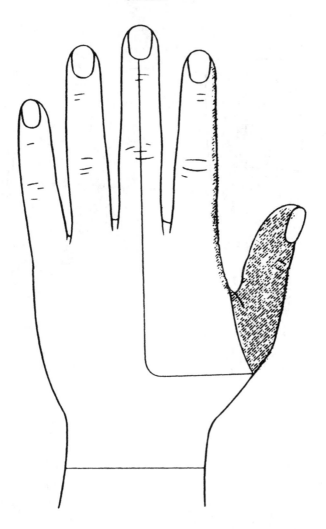

The Chicory zone located on the back of the left hand covers the thumb and the inner edge of the index finger. The zone extends from the inner edge of the index fingernail to the base of the thumb, running along the edge of the thumb toward its inner nail bed. The zones of the palm and the back of the hand meet on the sides of the fingers.

CHICORY

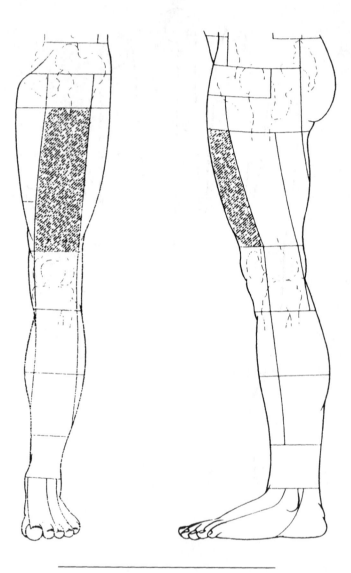

The Chicory zone on the left thigh begins on a horizontal line 1 finger width below the fold of the buttock and ends 1 finger width above the kneecap. The outside border at the zone's upper end aligns vertically with the front axial line; at its lower end the border lies 2 finger widths to the side of the kneecap. The inside border at the zone's upper end is 4 finger widths to the side of the midline; the inside border on the lower end is 1 finger width to the right of the kneecap.

CHICORY

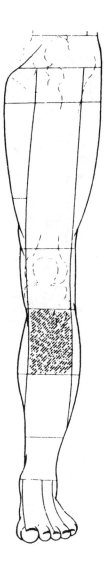

The Chicory zone on the left lower leg begins 3½ finger widths below the left kneecap and extends 6 finger widths downward. The side borders lie 2 finger widths to the left and right of the kneecap.

CHICORY

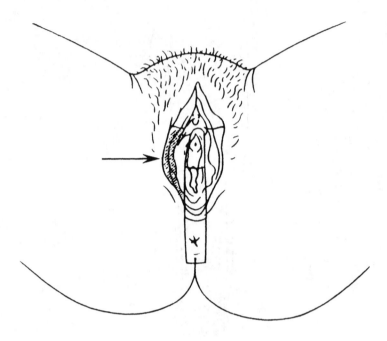

The Chicory flower also covers the outside of the right labia minora and the inside of the labia majora to the level of the clitoris.

CLEMATIS

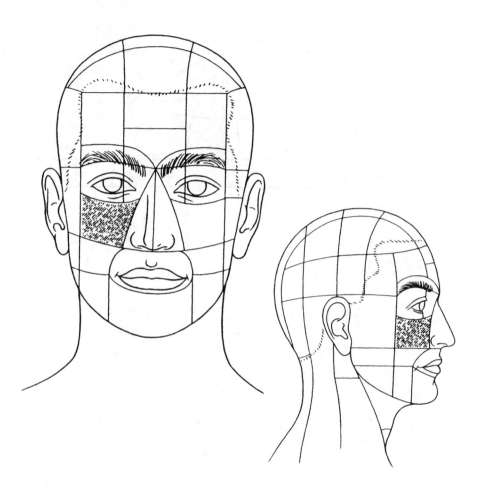

There are two Clematis zones on the neck and face. One zone begins at the level of the right orbit and ends on a horizontal line at the lower edge of the nose. The inside border begins approximately 3 mm from the nose. The outside border aligns vertically with the outer corner of the eyebrow.

CLEMATIS

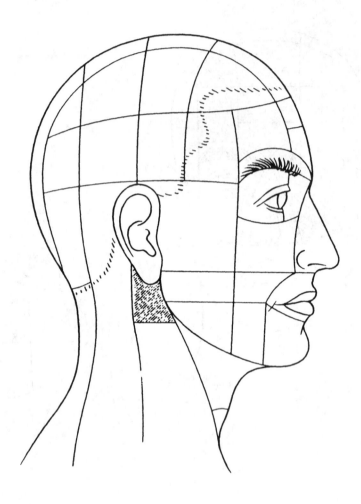

Another Clematis zone extends from the right ear downward to the angle of the jaw. The lateral borders align vertically with the front and rear edges of the ear.

CLEMATIS

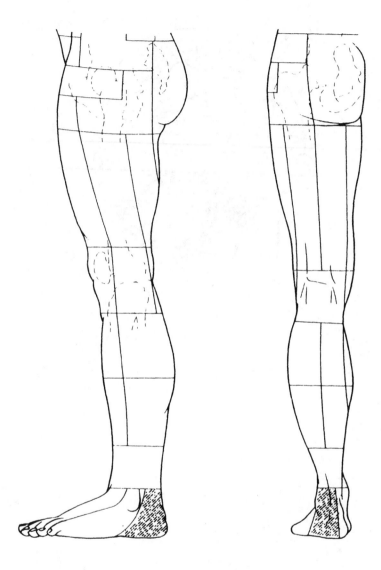

The third Clematis zone is located on the left foot in the area of the outer ankle bone. It aligns horizontally with the upper edge of the inner ankle bone and extends downward to the foot. The back border is formed by the Achilles tendon; the front border begins at the back edge of the outer ankle bone and slopes toward the front.

CRAB APPLE

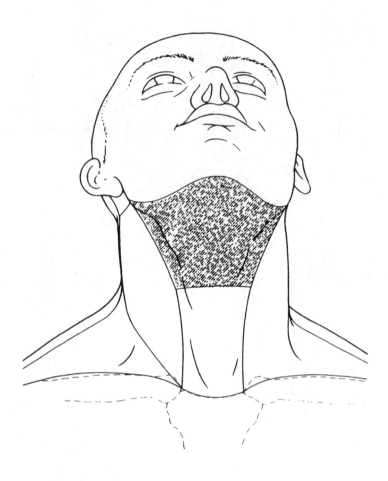

The Crab Apple zone begins at the lower edge of the chin and extends to the middle of the Adam's apple. The outer borders are formed by the upper edges of the sternocleidomastoid muscles.

CRAB APPLE

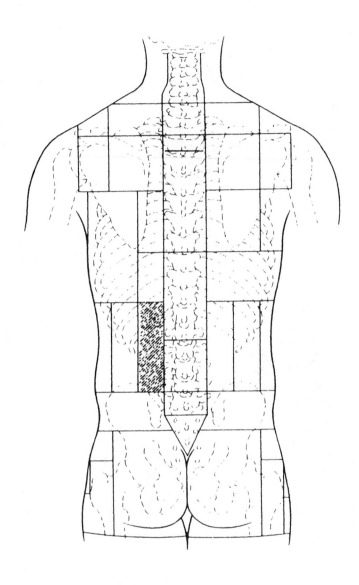

The Crab Apple zone on the back begins at the level of the eleventh thoracic vertebra and ends at the level of the fourth lumbar vertebra. Its inside border lies 2 finger widths to the left of the midline. The zone extends 3 finger widths to the left.

CRAB APPLE

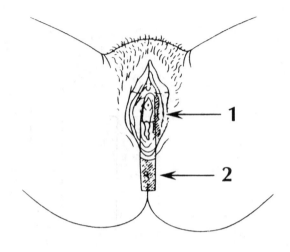

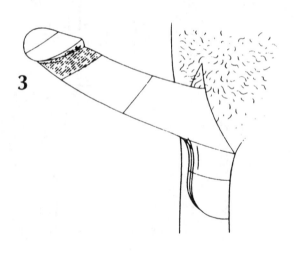

At the genitals, the Crab Apple zone for a woman covers the inside of the left labia minora (1) and the anus (2), extending to the point where the reddish color of the skin around the anus ends.

For a man, the Crab Apple zone begins at the shaft of the penis, near its tip (3), and extends approximately one finger width toward the scrotum. The Crab Apple zone also covers the anus, as described above.

ELM

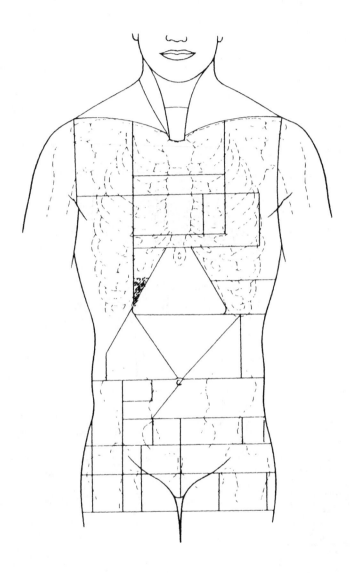

The Elm zone on the trunk begins 3 finger widths below the sternum and 4 finger widths to the right of the midline. The inside border of this zone follows the costal arch.

ELM

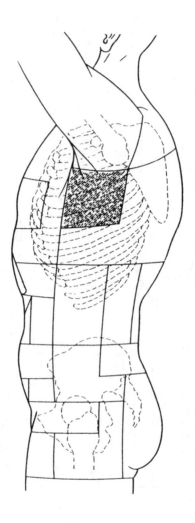

The Elm zone in the middle of the left armpit begins at the level of the fifth thoracic vertebra and ends at the level of the eighth thoracic vertebra. The outer borders align vertically with the front and back axial folds.

ELM

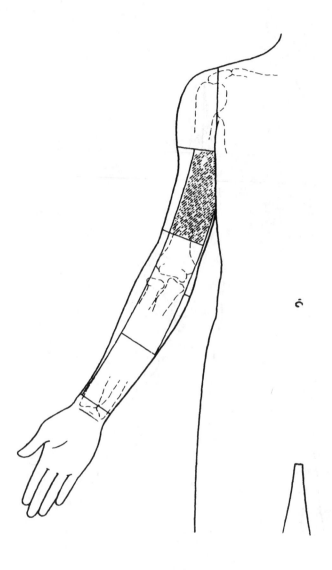

The Elm zone on the front side of the right upper arm begins 2 finger widths below the inner axial fold and ends 3 finger widths above the elbow fold. The outside border runs along the outer rim of the biceps; the inside border runs along the bicep's inner rim.

ELM

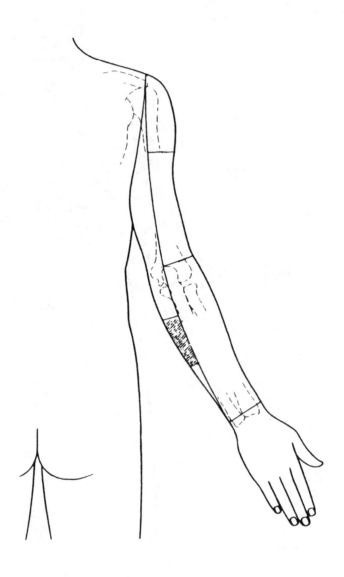

The Elm zone on the outside of the right arm begins 2 finger widths below the elbow and extends downward 5 finger widths. The inside border follows the line from the outer edge of the little finger to the inner fold of the elbow. The outer border runs along the edge of the ulna bone.

GENTIAN

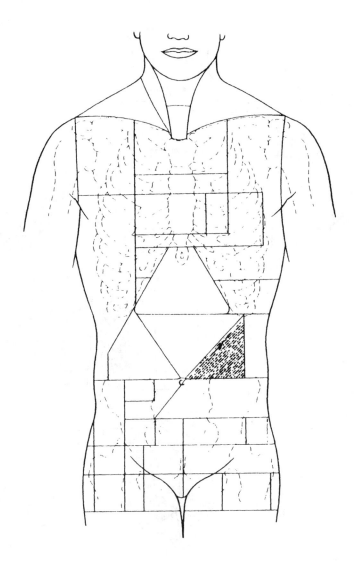

The Gentian zone on the trunk is located on the left side of the abdomen. Its lower border aligns horizontally with the navel and extends to the left to align vertically with the nipple line. The upper border begins at the midpoint of the tenth rib, running diagonally to the navel.

GENTIAN

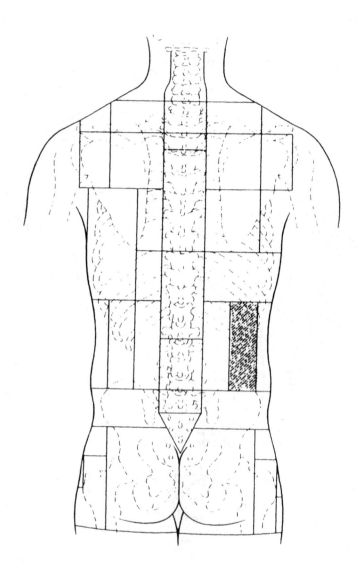

The Gentian zone on the back begins at the level of the eleventh thoracic vertebra and ends at the level of the fourth lumbar vertebra. The inner border is located approximately 5 finger widths to the right of the midline and extends 3 finger widths to the right.

GENTIAN

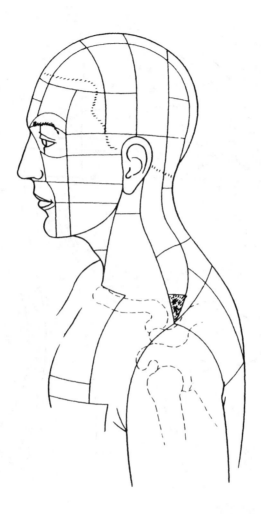

The Gentian zone on the left shoulder is located in a triangle formed by the frontward prominence of the trapezius muscle and the back edge of the muscle where it attaches to the spine of the scapula. The outer end point is the intersection of the extensions of the front and back axial folds upward, in an indentation that is often painful on palpation. The inner margin is about 1¹⁄₂ finger widths away.

GENTIAN

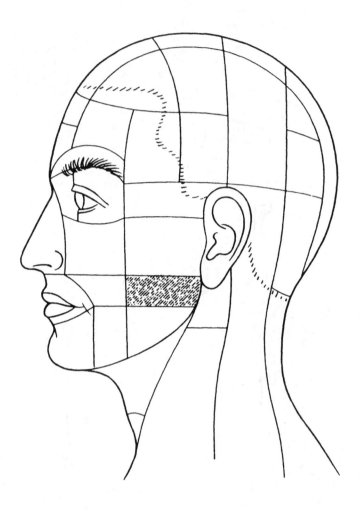

Another Gentian zone is located in the left facial hemisphere, beginning on a horizontal line with the bottom of the nose and ending in another horizontal line at the level with the corner of the mouth. The inside border aligns vertically with the outside corner of the left eyebrow and extends backward to end at the base of the earlobe.

GENTIAN

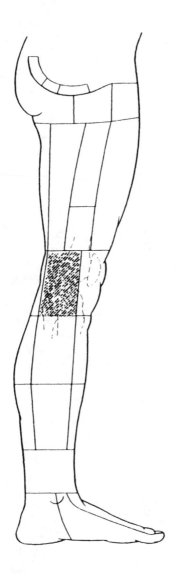

The Gentian zone on the inside of the left knee begins 2 finger widths to the inside of the kneecap and extends 4 finger widths toward the back. Its upper border aligns horizontally 1 finger width above the kneecap; its lower border aligns horizontally $3\frac{1}{2}$ finger widths below the kneecap.

GENTIAN

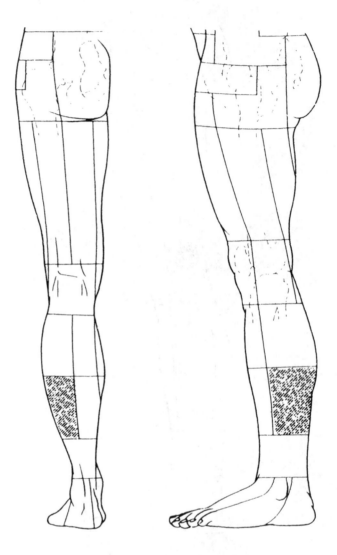

The Gentian zone on the left leg begins 4 finger widths above the upper edge of the left inner ankle bone and extends 6 finger widths upward. The back border is located in the middle of the calf, on an line running from the Achilles tendon to the middle of the knee. The front border lies on a vertical line 2 finger widths to the side of the kneecap.

GENTIAN

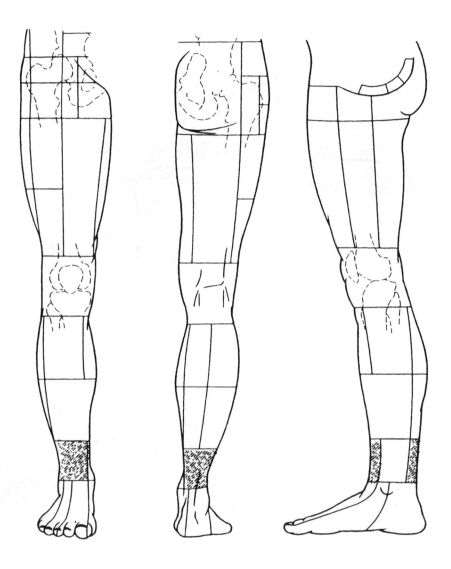

This Gentian zone on the right leg begins at the level of the inner ankle bone's upper edge and extends 4 finger widths upward. The front border aligns vertically with the front edge of the inner ankle bone. The zone extends around the front of the ankle and ends 1 finger width in back of the inner ankle bone.

GENTIAN

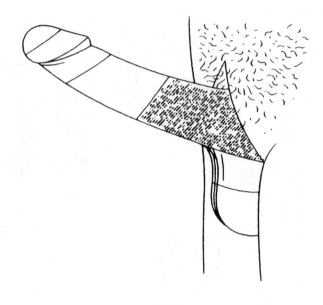

This Gentian zone, applicable to men only, begins halfway between the lower border of the Crab Apple zone (see page 94) and the base of the penis. The zone extends to the base of the penis.

Gorse

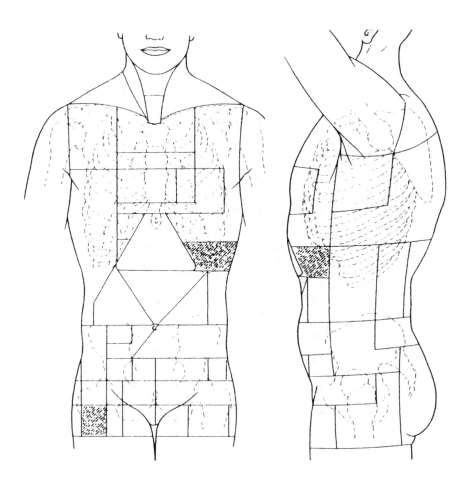

The Gorse flower is applicable to several zones on the body. The upper zone on the body's left side begins on a horizontal line equidistant between the navel and the sternum. The zone extends 3 finger widths upward. The inside border aligns with the costal arch; the ouside border aligns vertically with the axial fold.

The lower Gorse zone on the body's right side begins at the level of the pubic bone and ends 1 finger width below the level of the fold of the buttock. The inside border aligns vertically with the nipple. The outside border aligns with the front axial fold.

GORSE

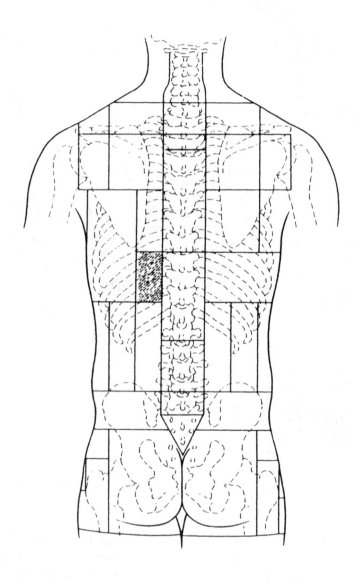

The Gorse zone on the back begins at the level of the eighth thoracic vertebra and ends at the level of the eleventh thoracic vertebra. The inside border is 2 finger widths to the side of the midline of the back; from there the zone extends 3 finger widths to the left.

GORSE

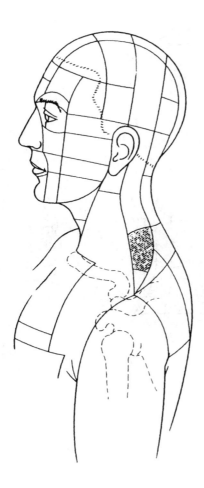

This Gorse zone on the left side extends from the frontal prominence of the trapezius muscle to its thicker aspect extending off the spine of the scapula. The inner border is formed by the base of the neck; the zone extends laterally to the outer one-third of the clavicle and spine of the scapula.

GORSE

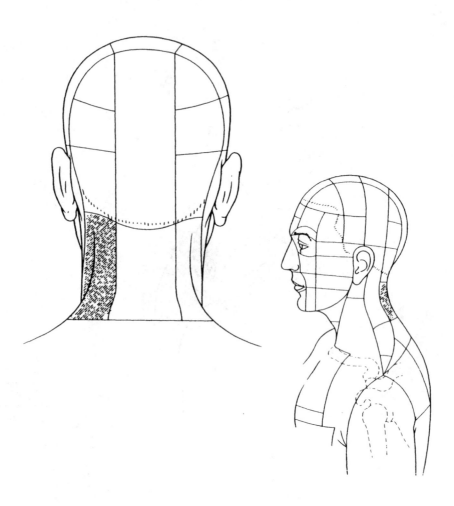

The Gorse zone on the left side of the neck begins at the base of the skull and ends at the base of the neck. The left border lies 2 finger widths behind the back of the ear and extends downward. The right border is 1½ finger widths to the side of the midline of the neck.

GORSE

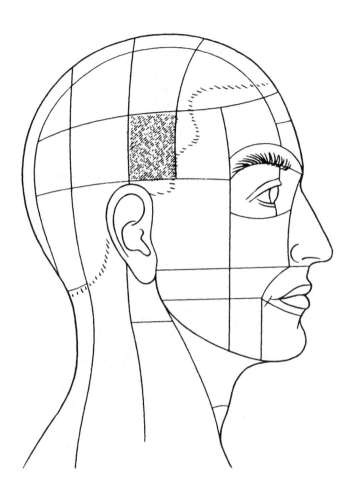

The Gorse zone on the right side of the head aligns horizontally with the top of the ear and extends 3 finger widths upward. The front border lies on a vertical line 2½ finger widths behind the outer edge of the eyebrow. The back border aligns vertically with the tip of the ear.

GORSE

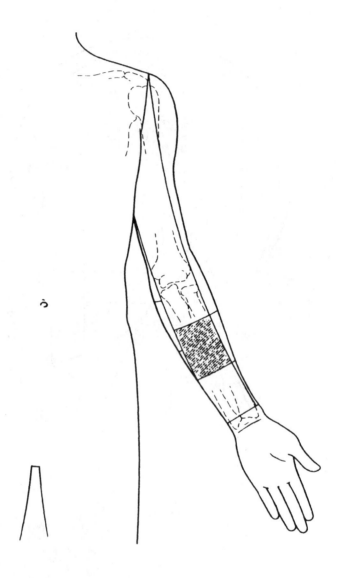

The Gorse zone located on the inside of the left arm begins 3 finger widths below the fold of the elbow and ends 5 finger widths below that. The inside border lies on a line from the outer edge of the little finger to the inner elbow fold. The outside border lies along the edge of the radius.

GORSE

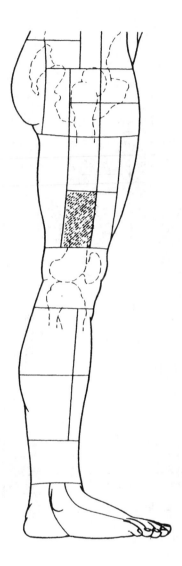

The Gorse zone located on the outside of the right thigh begins 1 finger width above the kneecap and extends 6 finger widths upward. The left border lies on a vertical line 2 finger widths to the side of the kneecap; the zone extends 4 finger widths toward the back.

HEATHER

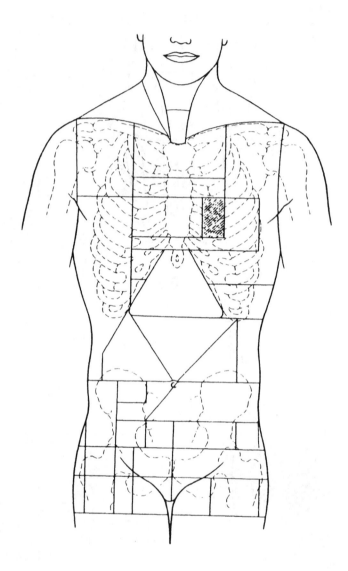

The Heather zone stretches from the third to the sixth intercostal space on the left side of the chest. The inside border begins 2 finger widths to the left of midline and extends 2 finger widths to the left.

HEATHER

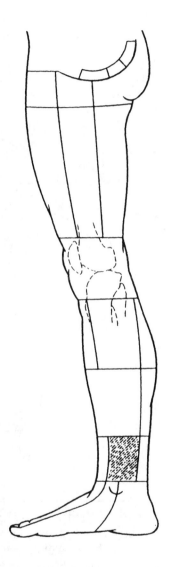

The Heather zone on the right leg begins at the upper corner of the inner ankle bone and extends 4 finger widths upward. The front border aligns vertically with the front edge of the inner ankle bone; the back border is 1 finger width behind the inner ankle bone's back edge.

HOLLY

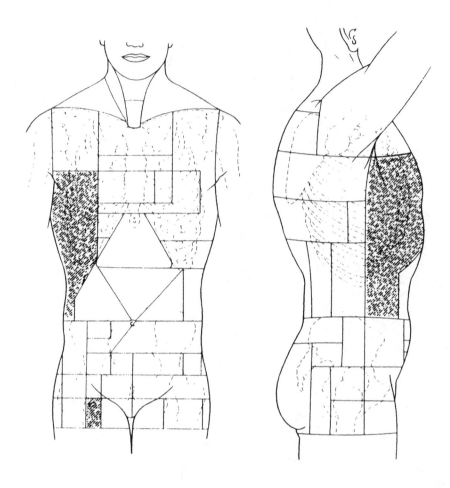

The upper Holly zone begins at the third intercostal area, approximately 4 finger widths to the right of midline. It runs on the right side from the axial fold downward, ending at the level of the navel. The front border extends downward to the costal arch. From there it runs along the costal arch to the palpable end of the eleventh rib, and then continues down in a straight line.

The lower Holly zone begins at the level of the pubic bone and ends 1 finger width below an imaginary line from the buttock's fold to the front. The inner edge lies 4 finger widths to the right of the midline; the zone extends 2 finger widths to the right.

HOLLY

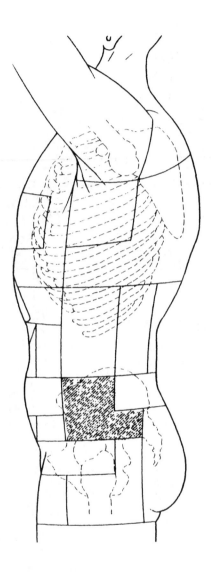

The Holly zone on the left side begins at the level of the fourth lumbar vertebra and extends to the level of the pubic bone. The front border aligns vertically with the front axial fold. The back border aligns vertically with the rear axial fold, extending four finger widths downward from the level of the navel. From there the zone extends 3 finger widths toward the back.

HOLLY

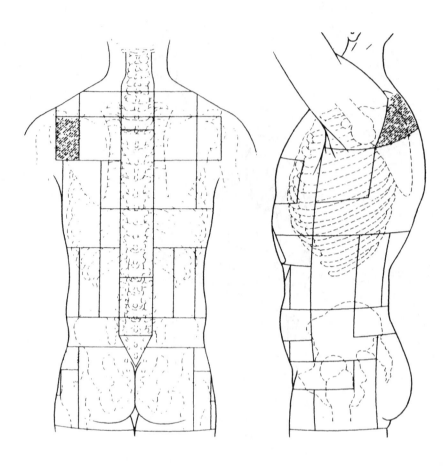

The Holly zone on the left side of the back begins at the level of the second thoracic vertebra and ends at the level of the fifth thoracic vertebra. The outer edge extends upward from the rear axial fold. The zone extends from the outer border 3 finger width to the right.

HOLLY

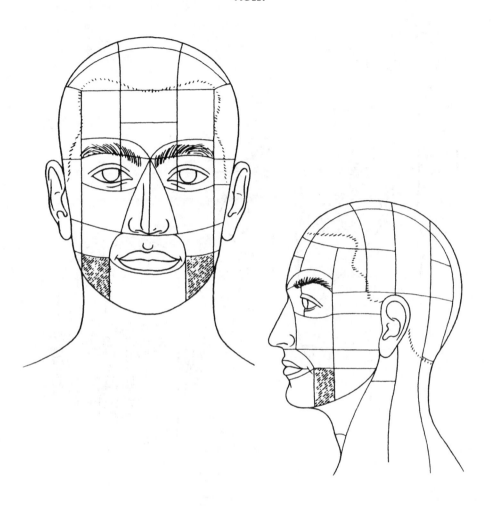

The Holly flower is applicable to two symmetrical zones that begin horizontal to the corners of the mouth and end at the jaw line. The front borders align vertically with the corners of the mouth. The back borders align vertically with the outer corners of the eyebrows.

HOLLY

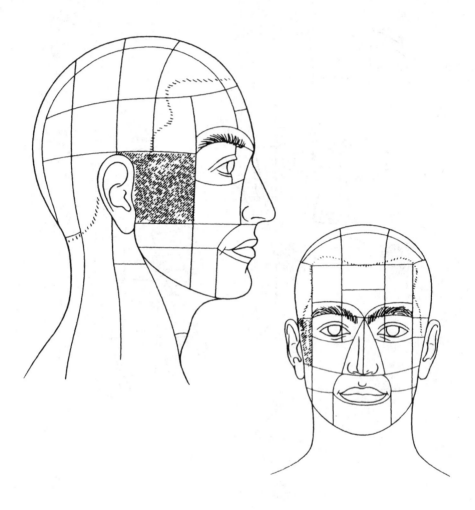

This Holly zone extends horizontally from the outer corner of the right eyebrow and ends horizontal to the bottom of the nose. The inner border aligns vertically with the outer corner of the eyebrow. The outer border is at the right edge of the ear.

HOLLY

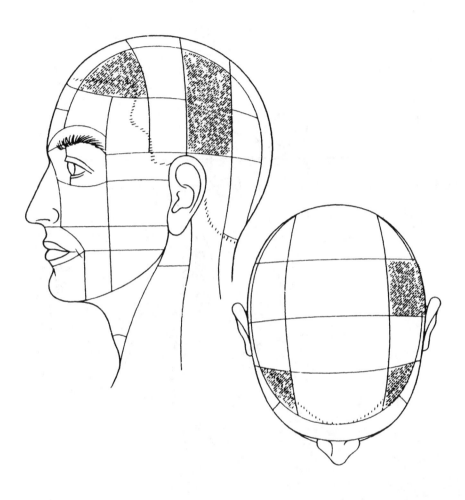

There are four Holly zones on the head: two frontal zones, one zone on the back left side, and one zone on the back right side. The two frontal zones begin on vertical lines 1½ finger widths to the left and right of the head's midline and extend 3 finger widths to the sides. The front border is marked by the hairline; the back border lies 3 finger widths behind the front.

The back zone on the left side of the head begins 1½ finger widths to the left of the midline and ends horizontal to the tip of the ear. The front border aligns vertically with the tip of the ear. The zone extends 3 finger widths to the back.

HOLLY

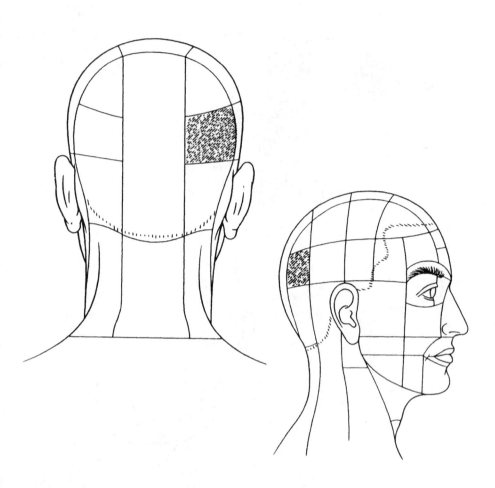

The Holly zone on the right side of the head begins 3 finger widths behind the tip of the right ear and extends 3 finger widths toward the back. The upper border lies 3 finger widths above.

HOLLY

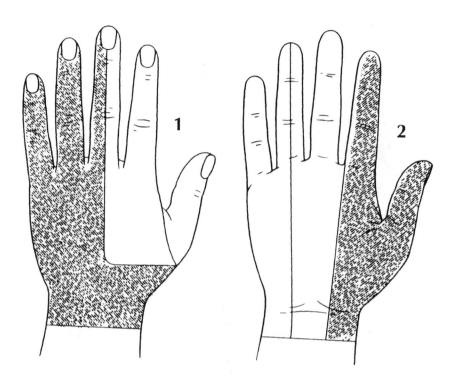

The Holly flower applies to zones on both the back of the left hand and the palm of the right hand. The zone on the back of the left hand (1) extends from a horizontal line 1 finger width above the wrist to the last three fingertips. The inside border is formed by a vertical line through the middle of the middle finger that extends downward to 2 finger widths above the wrist and runs across to the base of the thumb. The outside border runs along the outer edge of the hand to the outside of the little finger.

The zone located on the inside of the right hand (2) extends from a horizontal line 1 finger width above the wrist to the tips of the index finger and thumb. The right border runs along the outer edge of the wrist to the corner of the thumbnail. The left border begins 1 finger width inside the right edge of the wrist and continues to the left side of the index finger.

HOLLY

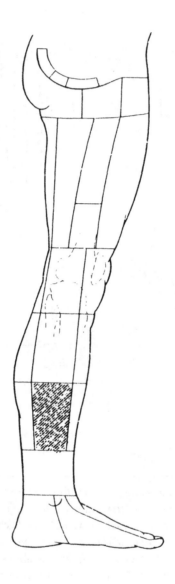

The Holly zone on the left leg begins 4 finger widths above the left inner ankle bone and extends 6 finger widths upward. The front border lies on the inner rim of the shin and extends 4 finger widths to the back. The zone narrows toward its lower edge, the back border lying 3 finger widths from the front.

HOLLY

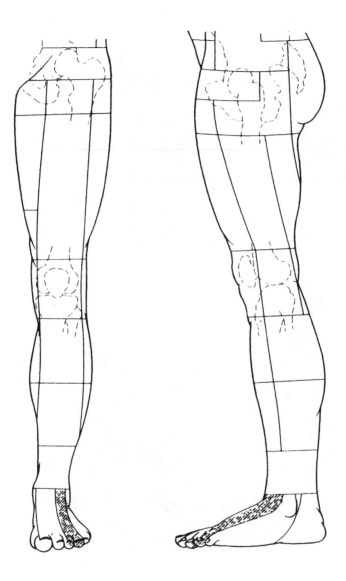

The Holly zone on the left foot begins at the level of the inner ankle bone's upper edge and extends toward the toes. The inside border runs through the midline of the foot to the middle of the middle toe. The outside border begins at the front of the outer ankle bone and extends to the space between the fourth and fifth toes. The zone ends at the beginning of the sole of the foot.

HOLLY

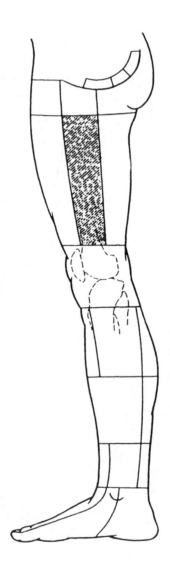

The Holly zone on the inside of the right thigh begins on a horizontal line 1 finger width below the fold of the buttock and ends 1 finger width above the kneecap. The back border lies on the body's medial line. The upper part of the zone extends 4 finger widths toward the front, tapering to a distance of 2½ finger widths above the kneecap.

HOLLY

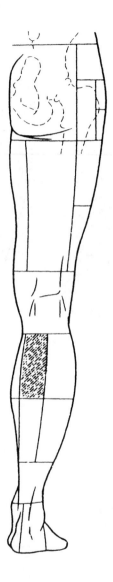

The Holly zone on the back of the right lower leg begins 3½ finger widths below the fold of the knee and extends 6 finger widths downward. The back border lies in the middle of the calf on a vertical line from the Achilles tendon to the middle of the knee. The zone extends 3 finger widths to the inside.

127

HOLLY

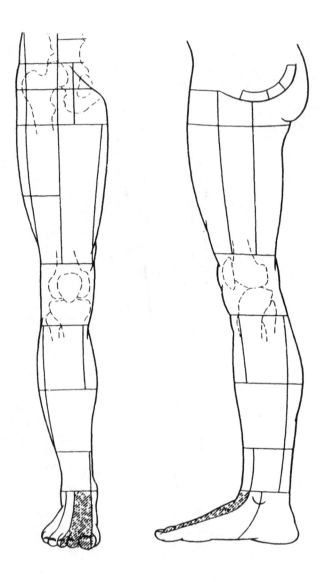

The Holly zone on the right foot begins at the top of the inner ankle bone and extends downward to the tips of the toes, ending at the beginning of the sole of the foot. The inside edge runs from the front of the ankle bone to the outside corner of the big toe. The outside edge runs from the middle of the foot to the middle of the middle toe. The lower border is located on the beginning of the sole; the inside of the toes belong to this zone.

HOLLY

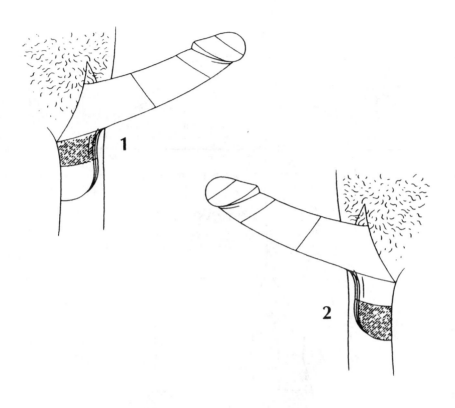

Finally, there is a Holly zone that covers the upper half of the right testicle (1). The zone begins on the midline and ends at the base of the testicle. The Holly flower also applies to the lower half of the left testicle (2). The zone begins on the midline and ends at the bottom of the testicle.

HONEYSUCKLE

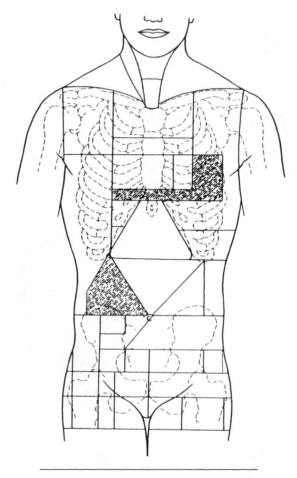

The Honeysuckle flower covers two zones on the trunk of the body. The upper zone on the left begins at the third intercostal space and extends to the seventh. The outside border of this zone is located 8 finger widths to the left of midline. The zone extends 4 finger widths to the right, toward the midline. Below this section, at the width of approximately 1¹/₂ fingers, the zone extends across the midline 4 finger widths to the right of the sternum.

The Honeysuckle zone on the lower right side has points of origin at the navel and at the inside angle of the tenth rib. The zone extends diagonally from the tenth rib to the navel. The outside border runs diagonally outward along the ridge of the floating ribs, then vertically downward from the outer border of the ribs to the level of the navel.

HONEYSUCKLE

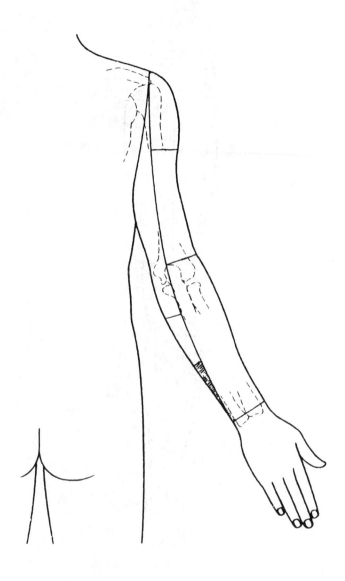

The Honeysuckle zone on the back of the right arm begins 6 finger widths below the fold of the elbow and ends 1 finger width above the wrist. The inside border lies on a line running from the outer edge of the little finger toward the inner elbow fold. The outside border runs along the edge of the ulna.

HONEYSUCKLE

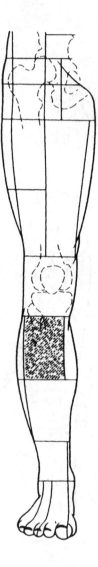

The zone on the front side of the right leg begins 3¹/₂ finger widths below the kneecap and extends 6 finger widths downward. The right border lies 2 finger widths to the right of the kneecap. The left border aligns vertically with the left edge of the kneecap.

HORNBEAM

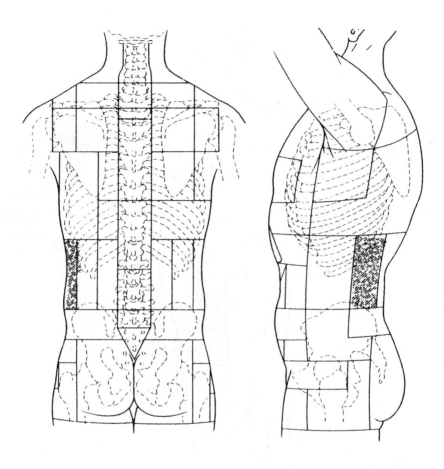

The Hornbeam zone on the left side of the back begins at the level of the eleventh thoracic vertebra and ends at the level of the fourth lumbar vertebra. The outside border aligns vertically with the rear axial fold; the zone extends 3 finger widths toward the spine.

HORNBEAM

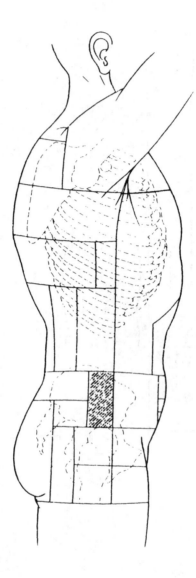

The Hornbeam zone on the right side of the body begins at the iliac crest and ends at the level of the pubic hair line. The front border aligns vertically with the front axial fold. The zone extends from the front border 3½ finger widths toward the spine.

HORNBEAM

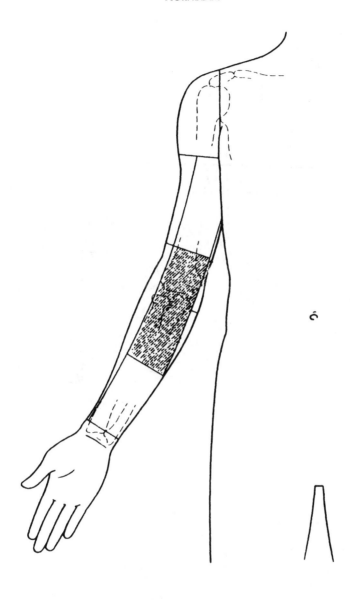

The Hornbeam zone on the inside of the right arm begins 3 finger widths above the fold of the inner arm and ends 6 finger widths below the arm fold. The outside edge runs along the outer rim of the lower biceps muscle toward the thumb. The inside edge extends along the inner rim of the lower biceps muscle toward the little finger.

IMPATIENS

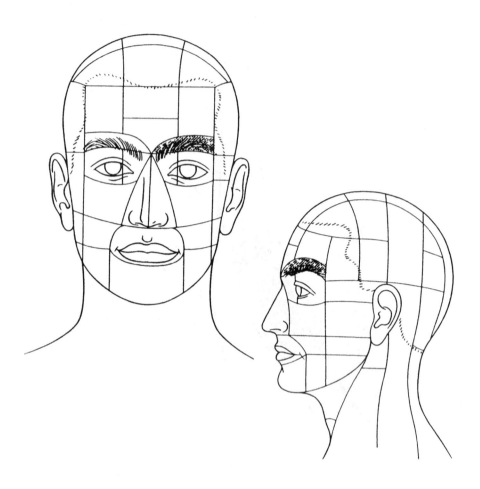

The Impatiens flower covers the zone of the left eyebrow.

IMPATIENS

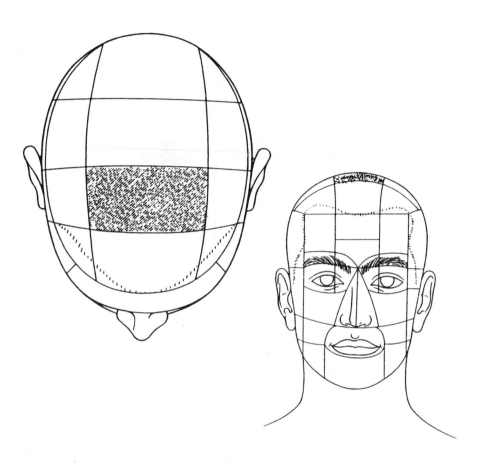

The Impatiens zone on the head begins 3 finger widths above the hairline and on a line extending from the tips of the ears. The zone extends 1¹/₂ finger widths to the left and the right of the head's midline.

IMPATIENS

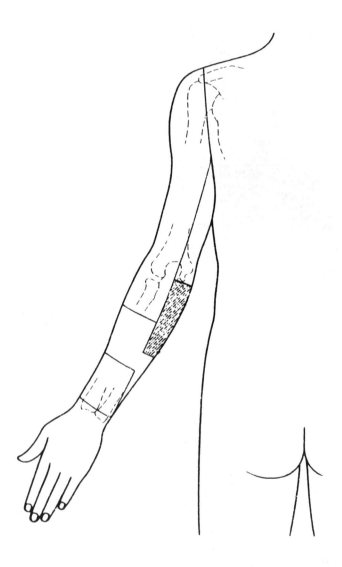

The Impatiens zone on the back side of the left arm begins at the tip of the elbow and extends 7 finger widths downward. One side border aligns vertically with the outer edge of the little finger and runs to the elbow fold. The other side border is located on the bony ridge of the ulna.

IMPATIENS

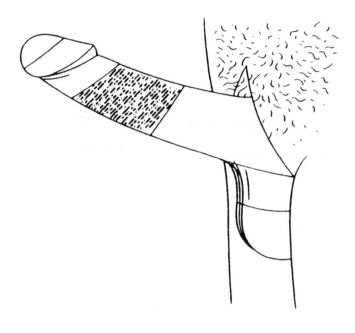

This Impatiens zone begins 1 finger width below the glans and extends half the distance toward the base of the penis, where it abuts the Gentian zone (see page 106).

LARCH

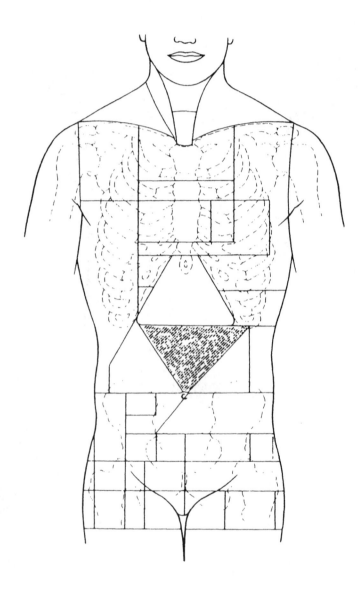

The Larch zone on the trunk begins on a horizontal line that is equidistant between the navel and the sternum. The left border aligns vertically with the nipple; the right border lies 1 finger width inside the inner edge of the ribs. The zone extends from these points downward to the navel.

LARCH

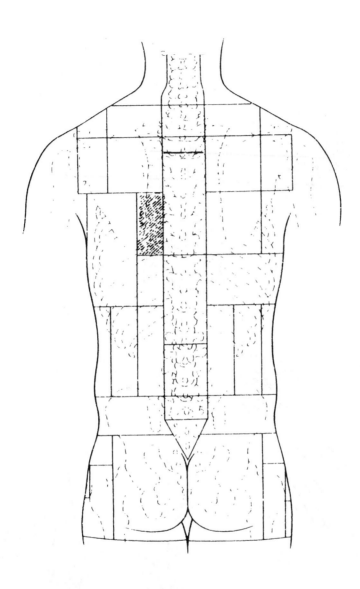

The Larch zone on the back begins at the level of the fifth thoracic vertebra and ends at the level of the eighth thoracic vertebra. The inside border lies 2 finger widths to the left of the midline of the back. The zone extends 3 finger widths to the left.

LARCH

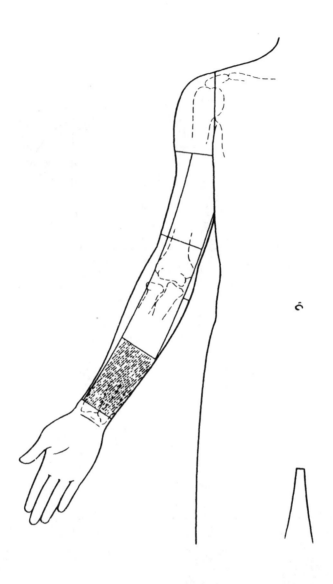

The Larch zone on the inside of the right arm begins 6 finger widths below the elbow fold and ends 1 finger width above the wrist. The inside border extends on a line from the outer edge of the little finger toward the inner elbow fold. The outside border is marked by the bony ridge of the radius bone.

Larch

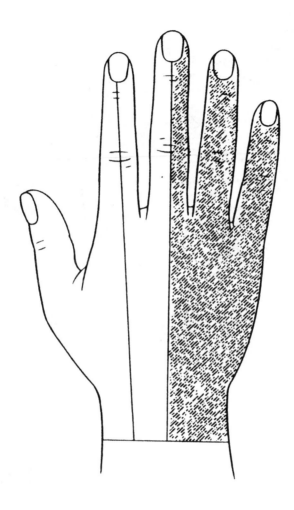

The Larch zone on the back of the right hand extends from 1 finger width above the wrist to the fingertips. The inside border runs from the middle of the wrist to the middle of the middle finger. The outside border lies on the outer edge of the hand and extends to the corner of the little finger.

LARCH

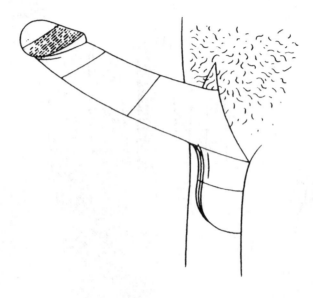

The Larch zone at the penis corresponds with the bottom half of the glans.
The zone ends at the upper edge of the rim of the glans.

MIMULUS

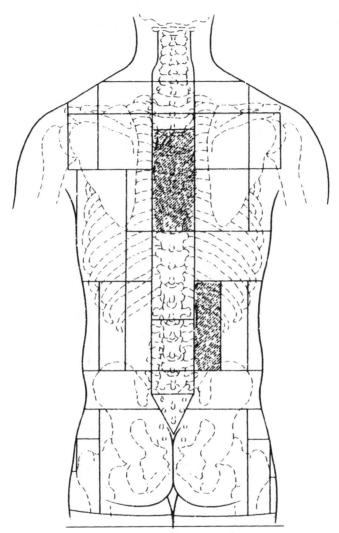

There are two Mimulus zones on the back. The upper zone begins at the level of the third thoracic vertebra and ends at the level of the eighth thoracic vertebra. The side borders are 2 finger widths each to the left and right of the midline.

The lower zone on the right side of the back begins at the level of the eleventh thoracic vertebra and ends at the level of the fourth lumbar vertebra. The inside border is 2 finger widths to the right of the midline. The zone extends 3 finger widths to the right.

MIMULUS

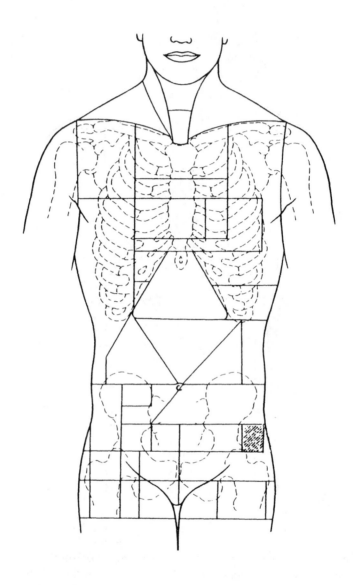

The Mimulus zone on the left side of the body aligns vertically with the left nipple on one side and the front axial fold on the other. The upper border lies on a horizontal line equidistant between the pubic crest and the navel. The lower border lies on a horizontal line 1 finger width above the pubic crest.

Mimulus

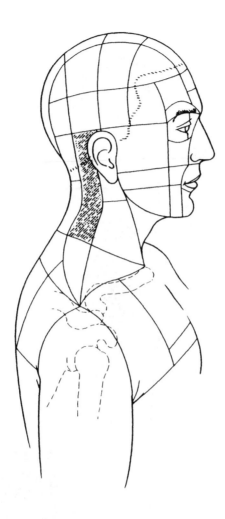

The Mimulus zone on the right side of the neck begins at the level of the tip of the ear and ends at the base of the neck. The front border aligns with the base of the ear; from there the zone extends 2 finger widths to the back.

MIMULUS

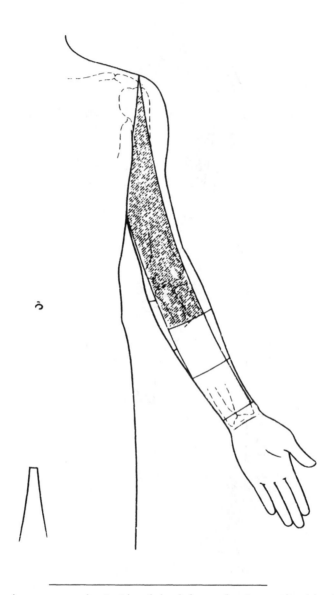

The Mimulus zone on the inside of the left arm begins at shoulder level, where the front axial extension intersects with the extension of the outer ridge of the biceps muscle. This palpable indentation is often painful to the touch. The zone ends 3 finger widths below the elbow fold. The outside border follows the outer ridge of the biceps muscle, and the inside border follows the inside ridge of the biceps muscle.

MIMULUS

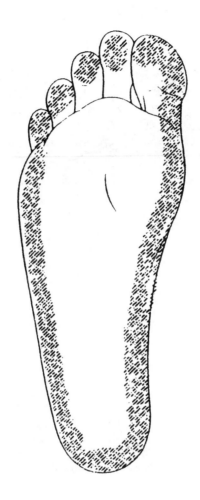

The Mimulus flower covers the entire sole of the right foot, including the bottoms of the toes.

MIMULUS

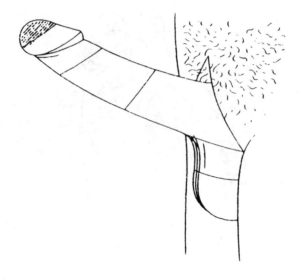

The Mimulus flower also covers the top half of the glans of the penis.

MUSTARD

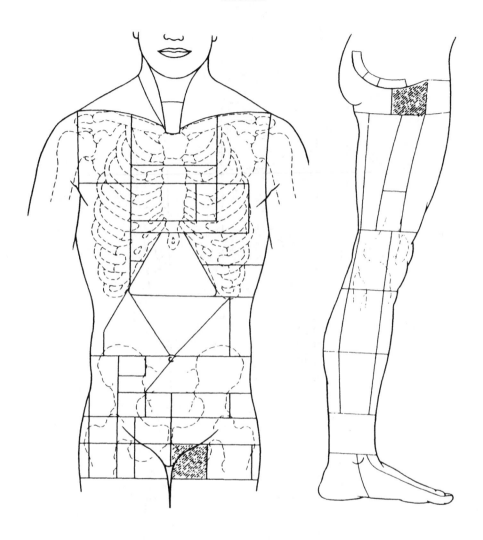

The Mustard zone located on the left side of the groin begins at the lower edge of the pubic bone and ends 1 finger width below an extension of the buttock's fold to the front. The zone encompasses the genitals. The inside border of this zone lies along the body's midline. The zone extends 4 finger widths to the left.

MUSTARD

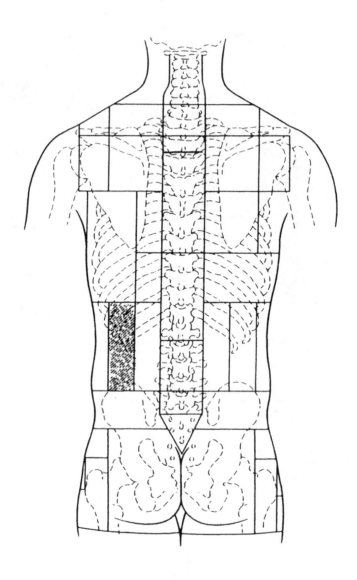

The Mustard zone on the back begins at the level of the eleventh thoracic vertebra and ends at the level of the fourth lumbar vertebra. The inside border lies 5 finger widths to the left of the midline. The zone extends laterally 3 finger widths.

MUSTARD

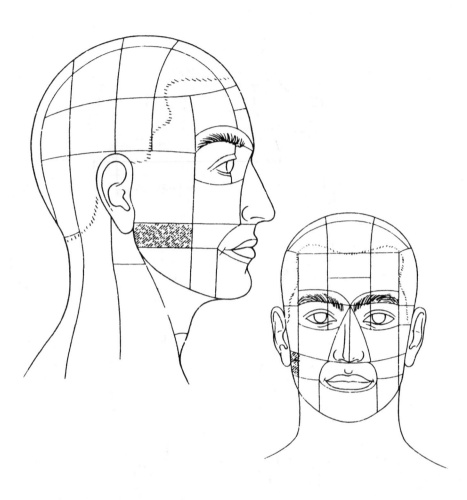

The Mustard zone on the right side of the face begins level with the bottom of the nose and ends level with the corner of the mouth. The inside border aligns vertically with the outside corner of the eyebrow; the outer border aligns with the earlobe.

MUSTARD

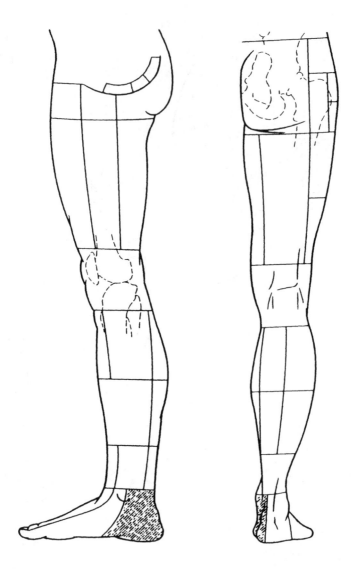

The Mustard zone on the right foot begins at the top of the inside ankle bone and ends at the bottom of the foot. The back border is formed by the Achilles tendon. The zone extends from the Achilles tendon over the ankle to the arch of the foot.

MUSTARD

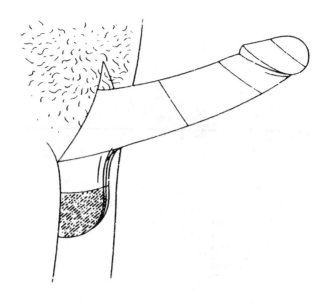

The Mustard flower applies to the lower half of the right testicle. The zone begins at the midline of the testicle and ends at the bottom of the testicle.

OAK

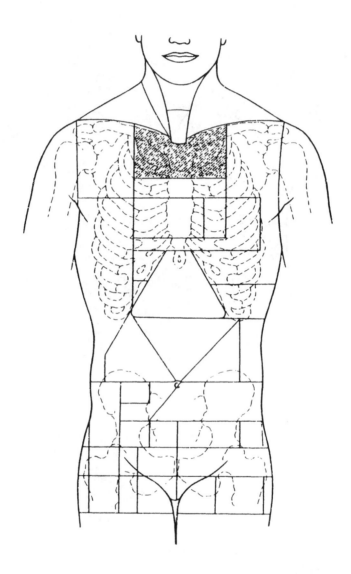

The Oak zone on the trunk begins at the upper prominence of the collarbone and ends about 1 finger width below in the second intercostal space. The outside borders lie 4 finger widths to the right and left of the midline.

OAK

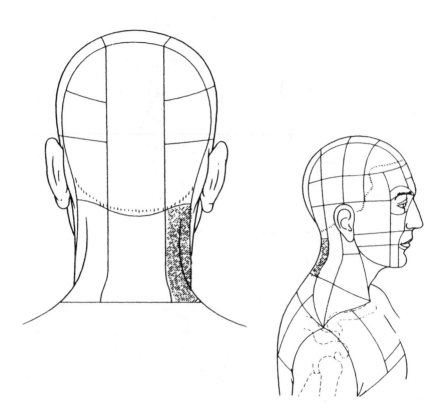

The Oak zone on the right side of the neck begins at the ridge of the skull. The front border is approximately 2 finger widths behind the back base of the ear and extends downward to the base of the neck. The back border lies 1¹/₂ finger widths to the right of the neck's midline.

OAK

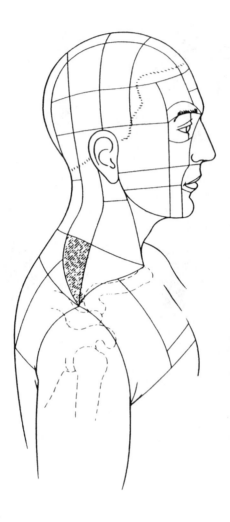

An adjoining Oak zone on the right side follows the front prominence of the trapezius muscle. The inside border of this zone aligns with the base of the neck; the outside border lies at the intersection of an extension from the front and back axial lines. This indentation is often painful when palpated.

OAK

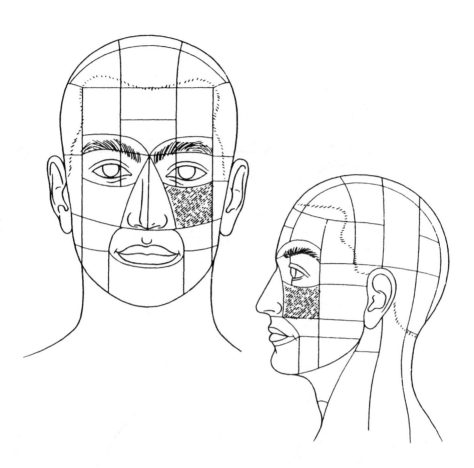

Another Oak zone begins at the level of the lower edge of the left eye socket and ends horizontal to the bottom of the nose. The zone sits approximately 3 mm from the side of the nose. The outside border aligns vertically with the outer corner of the left eyebrow.

OAK

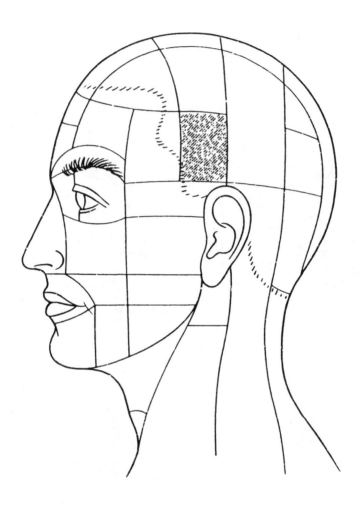

The Oak zone on the head aligns vertically with the tip of the ear, extending 3 finger widths upward. The front border begins 2½ finger widths behind the edge of the left eyebrow.

OAK

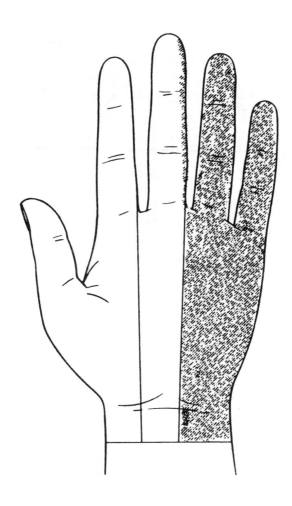

The Oak zone located on the palm side of the left hand extends from 1 finger width above the wrist to the tips of the outer fingers. The lateral border begins in the middle of the wrist and extends to the inside edge of the middle finger. The medial border runs along the outer edge of the hand to the outer corner of the little finger.

OAK

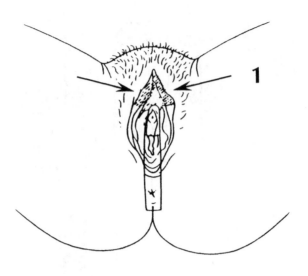

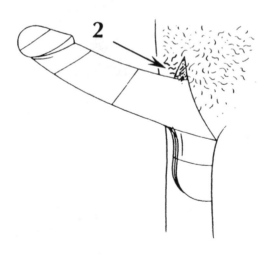

The Oak flower also applies to the genitals. The zone for women begins at the lower edge of the pubic bone and covers the inside of the labia majora, extending to the level of the tip of the clitoris (1). For men, the Oak zone begins at the lower margin of the pubic bone and extends in a triangle to the base of the penis (2).

OLIVE

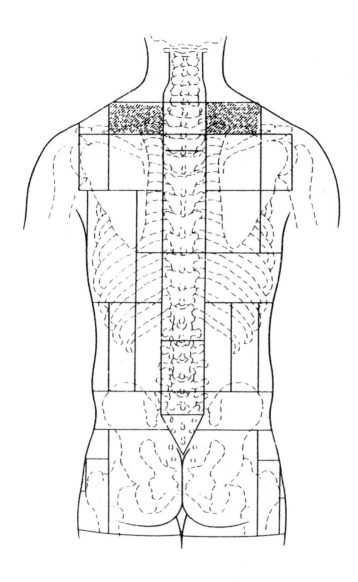

The Olive zone on the back covers areas to the left and right of the spine. The zone begins at the level of the sixth cervical vertebra at the upper border of the trapezius muscle and ends at the level of the second thoracic vertebra. The inside borders lie 2 finger widths to the left and the right of the back's midline; the zone extends 6 finger widths to the left and right.

OLIVE

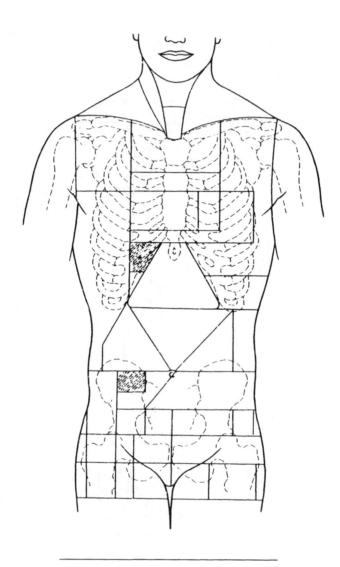

There are two Olive zones located on the right side of the trunk. The upper zone aligns horizontally with the lower part of the sternum and extends 3 finger widths downward. The inside border follows the costal arch; the outside border sits 4 finger widths to the side of midline.

The lower Olive zone on the trunk sits 3 finger widths to the right of the navel and aligns horizontally with it. The zone is 3 finger widths across and 2 finger widths high. The outside margin aligns vertically with the nipple.

OLIVE

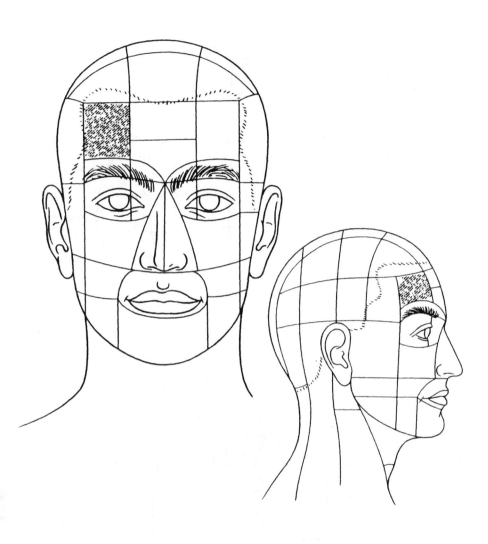

The Olive zone on the head begins at the hairline and extends above the right eyebrow. The inside border lies 1¹/₂ finger widths to the side of midline. The outside border aligns vertically with the outside corner of the eyebrow.

PINE

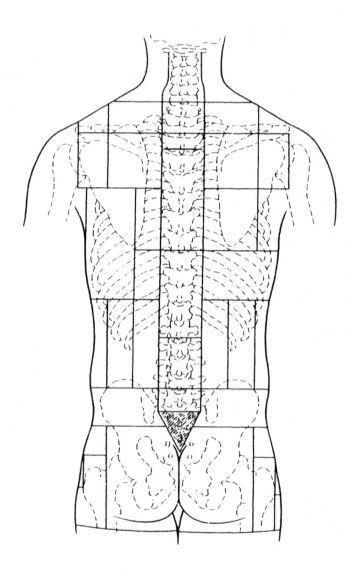

The Pine zone on the back begins at the upper rim of the sacrum. The zone extends 2 finger widths to the left and right of midline, sloping downward to the end of the anal fold.

PINE

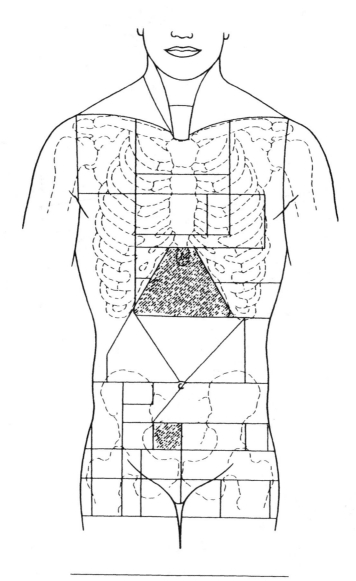

The Pine zone on the upper trunk begins at the lower end of the sternum, extending downward to a level equidistant between the lower sternum and the navel. The zone is bordered on both sides by the costal arch.

The lower Pine zone, located on the right side, begins at the midpoint between the pubis and the navel and ends at the level of the pubic hair line. The zone extends 3 finger widths to the right of midline.

PINE

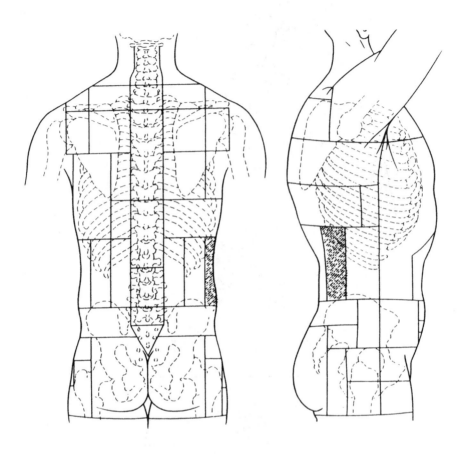

The Pine zone on the right side of the body begins at the level of the eleventh thoracic vertebra and ends at the level of the fourth lumbar vertebra. The zone aligns vertically with the back axial fold and extends 3 finger widths toward the spine.

PINE

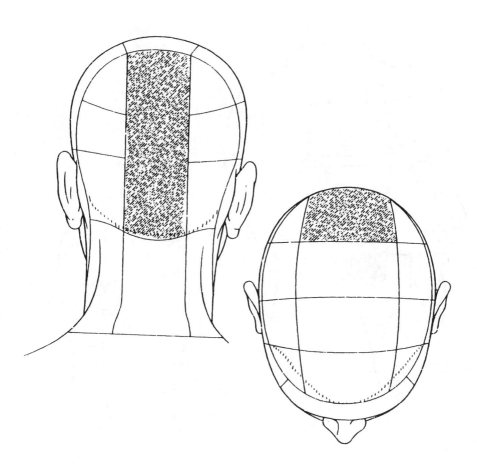

The Pine zone on the skull begins 3 finger widths behind the crown and ends at the occipital ridge. The zone extends 1½ finger widths to the left and right of the skull's midline.

PINE

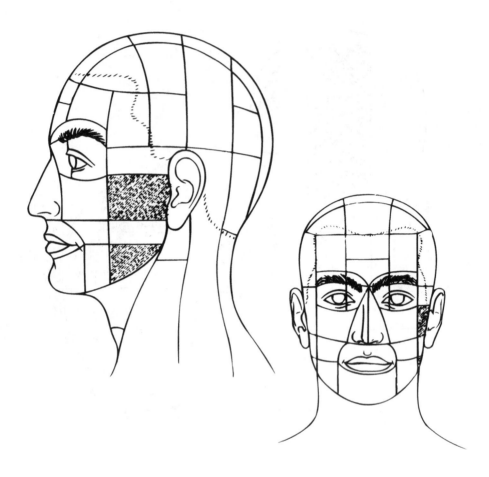

Pine also applies to two zones on the face. The upper zone begins horizontal to the lower rim of the left eye socket and ends horizontal to the bottom of the nose. The inside border aligns vertically with the outside corner of the eyebrow. The zone extends to the edge of the left ear.

The lower zone begins horizontal to the left corner of the mouth and ends on the lower ridge of the jaw. The front border aligns vertically with the outside corner of the eyebrow. The back zone extends toward the ear, ending at the ridge of the jawbone.

PINE

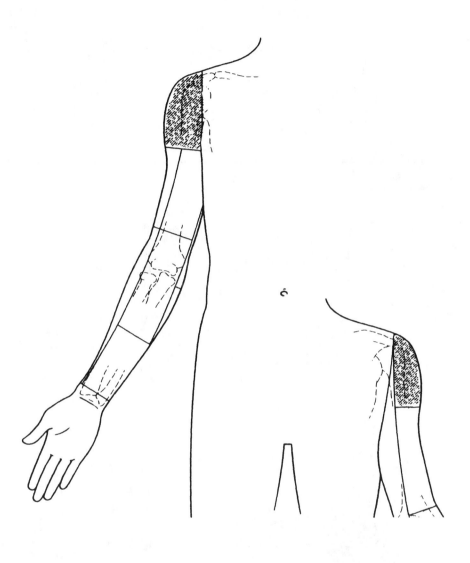

The Pine zone on the right upper arm begins at the edge of the shoulder in a palpable—often painful—indention found by following the front and back axial folds upward. The lower border of the zone aligns horizontally with the back axial line. The zone extends from the front axial line around the shoulder, ending 3 finger widths to the right of the back axial fold.

PINE

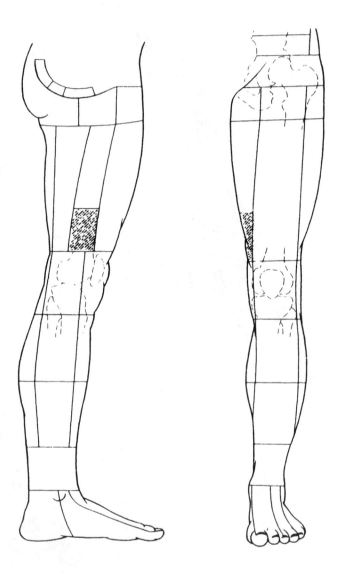

The Pine zone located on the left thigh begins 1 finger width above the kneecap and extends 4 finger widths above. The side border lies 1 finger width to the right of the kneecap, the zone extending 3 finger widths toward the inside of the thigh.

PINE

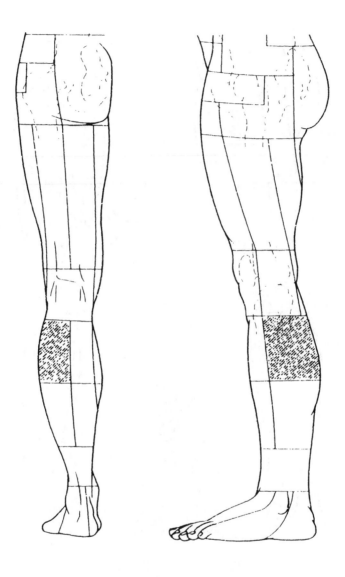

The Pine zone located on the left calf begins 3½ finger widths below the left kneecap and extends 6 finger widths downward. The back border runs through the middle of the calf, vertical to the Achilles tendon. The zone extends around the outside of the leg, ending 2 finger widths to the side of the kneecap.

PINE

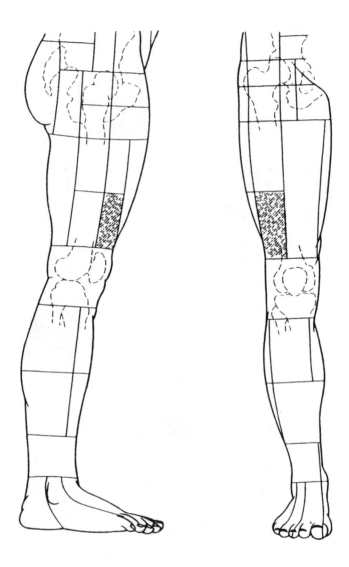

The Pine zone on the right thigh begins 1 finger width above the kneecap and extends 6 finger widths upward. The border in the front is located 2 finger widths to the inside of the femoral condyle, the bony protrusion at the side of the kneecap. The zone extends 3 finger widths to the side.

PINE

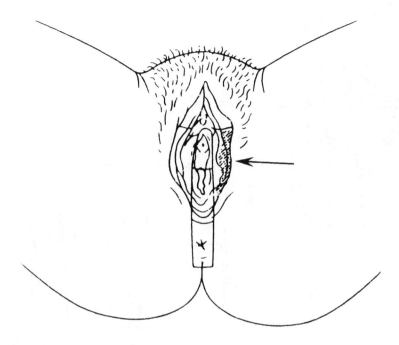

For women, Pine covers the inside of the left labia majora to the level of the clitoris, and the ouside of the labia minora.

RED CHESTNUT

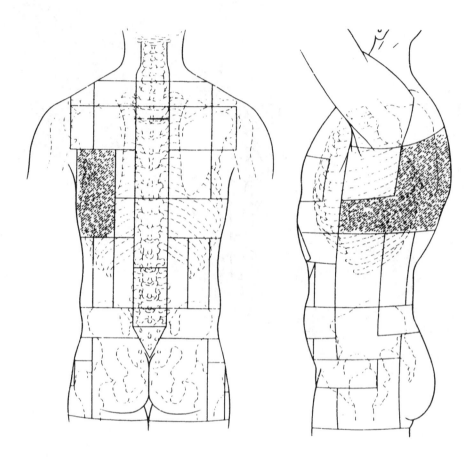

The Red Chestnut zone located on the left side of the body starts at the level of the fifth thoracic vertebra and ends at the level of the eleventh thoracic vertebra. The side border lies 5 finger widths from the midline, the zone extending to align vertically with the back axial fold, to the level of the eighth thoracic vertebra. The lower part of the zone continues around the side to align vertically with the front axial fold.

RED CHESTNUT

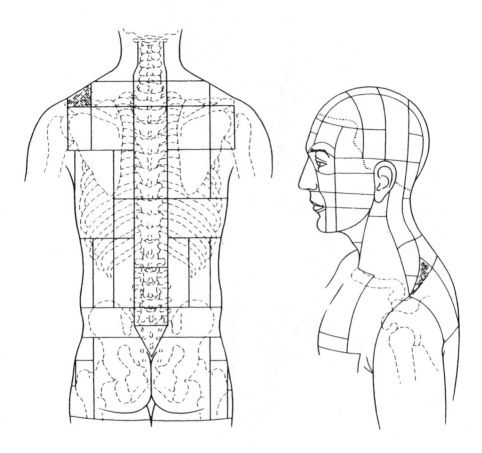

The Red Chestnut zone located on the left shoulder begins at the level of the sixth cervical vertebra. It follows the prominence of the trapezius muscle to the level of the second thoracic vertebra. The left border of the zone aligns vertically with the back axial fold. The zone extends 3 finger widths toward the spine.

RED CHESTNUT

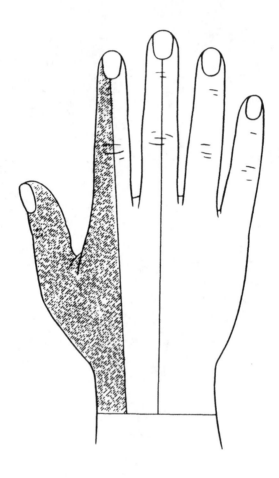

The Red Chestnut zone on the back of the right hand extends from 1 finger width above the wrist toward the thumb and index finger. The border on the thumb side extends to the corner of the thumbnail. The border on the index finger side begins 1 finger width to the side of the wrist fold and runs to the middle of the index finger.

ROCK ROSE

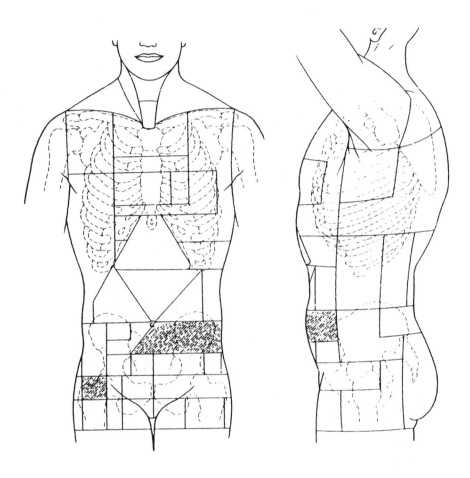

The Rock Rose zone on the left side of the trunk aligns horizontally with the navel and extends downward approximately 5 finger widths to the level of the anterior superior iliac spine. The medial border, extending 3 finger widths to the right of the midline at the bottom of the zone, slants diagonally to the navel. The lateral border of the zone aligns vertically with the front of the axial fold.

On the right side of the trunk the Rock Rose zone aligns horizon-tally approx-imately 2 finger widths above the upper edge of the pubic bone and extends downward to align with the lower edge of the pubic bone. The medial border aligns vertically with the right nipple; the lateral border aligns vertically with the front axial fold.

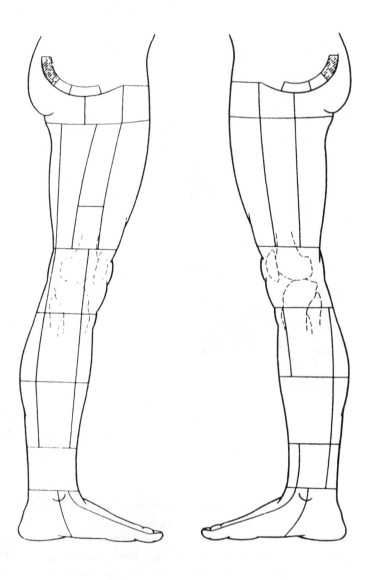

The Rock Rose zone that covers the tailbone begins above the anus, at the place where the red skin color around the anus ends, and extends upward to end at the anal fold. The zone is bordered on both sides by the buttocks.

ROCK ROSE

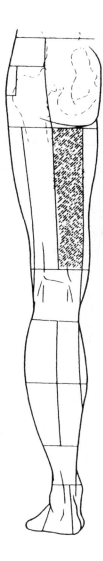

The Rock Rose zone on the back of the left thigh begins 1 finger width below the fold of the buttock and ends horizontal to a line 1 finger width above the kneecap. The left border is located on the midline of the thigh. At its lower end the zone extends 2½ finger widths to the right; at its upper end the zone extends 4 finger widths to the right.

ROCK ROSE

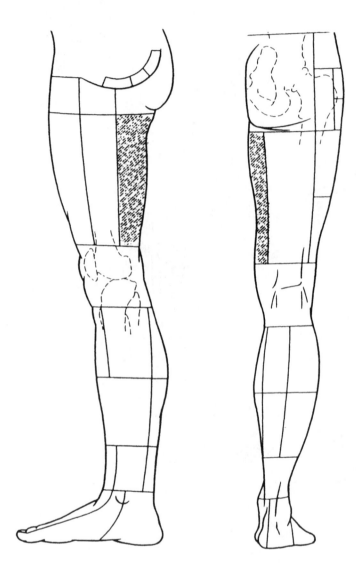

Another Rock Rose zone is located on the inside of the right thigh. It begins 1 finger width below the fold of the buttock and ends 1 finger width above the kneecap. The medial border lies 2½ finger widths to the left of the knee-cap. At its bottom the zone extends 2½ finger widths around the thigh toward the back. At its upper end the zone extends 4 finger widths toward the back.

ROCK ROSE

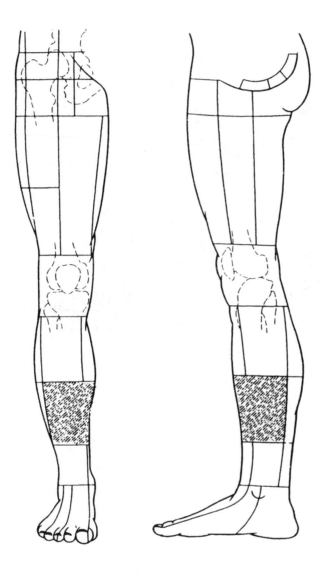

The Rock Rose zone located on the right shin begins 4 finger widths above the upper corner of the inside ankle bone and extends 6 finger widths upward. The lateral border aligns vertically 2 finger widths in front of the outer ankle bone. The zone extends around the shin to end 5 finger widths past the midline.

ROCK WATER

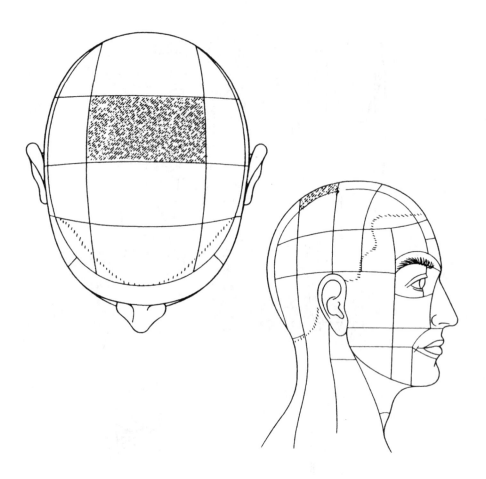

The Rock Water zone on the head begins at the crown and extends 3 finger widths toward the back of the skull. The side borders of this zone are 1¹/₂ finger widths to the right and left of the midline.

ROCK WATER

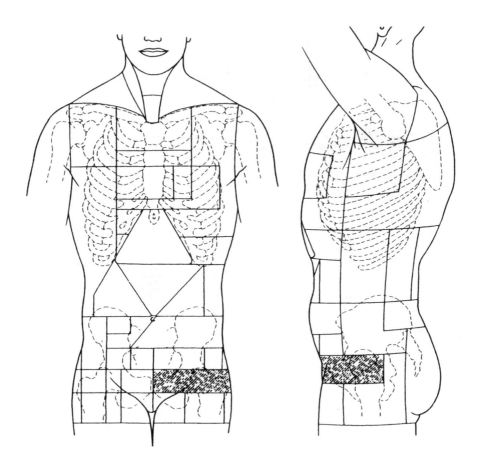

This Rock Water zone, located on the left side of the body, begins one finger width above the upper pubic bone and extends to the lower edge of the pubic bone. The zone extends from the midline across the left side, aligning vertically on the lateral side with the back axial fold.

ROCK WATER

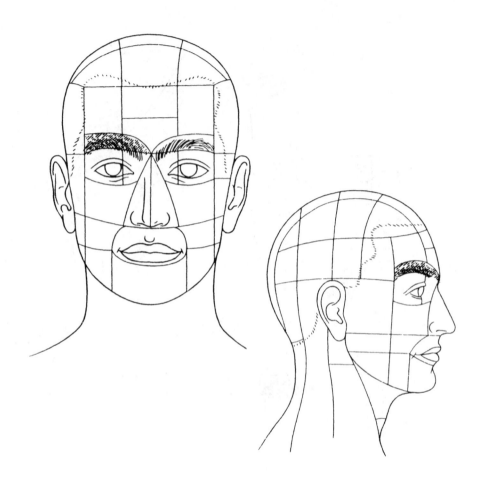

The Rock Water zone covers the entire right eyebrow.

ROCK WATER

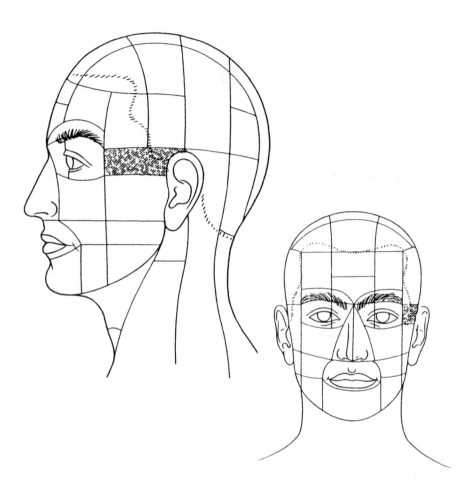

This zone on the left facial hemisphere begins at the corner of the left eyebrow and extends downward to align horizontally with the lower margin of the eye socket. The zone extends around the left side of the face to end at the edge of the left ear.

ROCK WATER

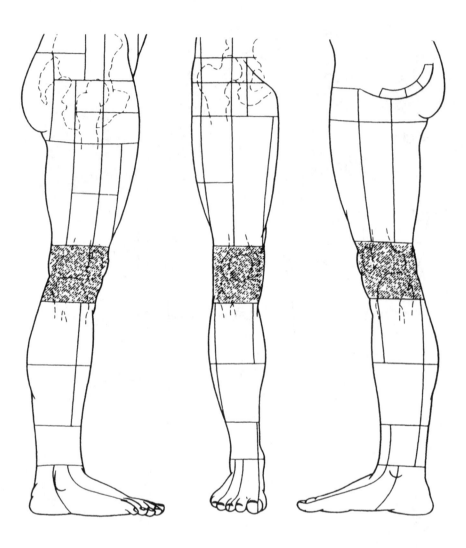

The Rock Water remedy applies to the entire right knee—front, side, and back. Its upper border lies 1 finger width above the kneecap; the lower border lies 3½ finger widths below the kneecap.

SCLERANTHUS

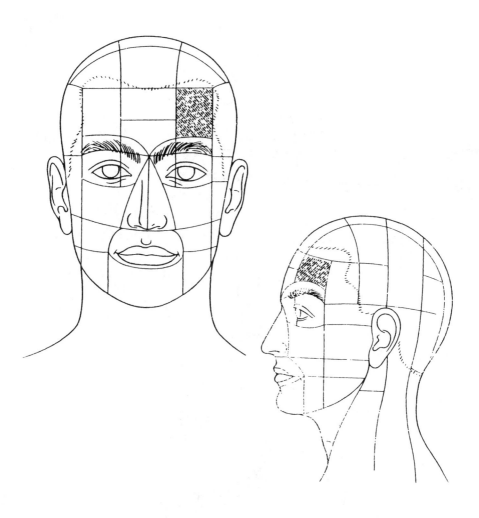

The Scleranthus zone on the face begins on the left at the hairline and ends just above the left eyebrow. The inside border is located 1½ finger widths to the side of the facial midline; the outside border aligns vertically with the end of the eyebrow.

SCLERANTHUS

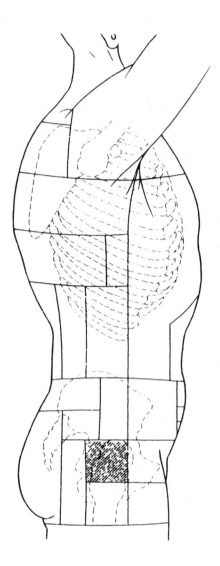

At the pelvis, the Scleranthus zone is located on the right side, aligning vertically with the front and back axial folds. The upper border lies 1 finger width above the hip socket; the lower border lies 1 finger width below the tailbone.

STAR OF BETHLEHEM

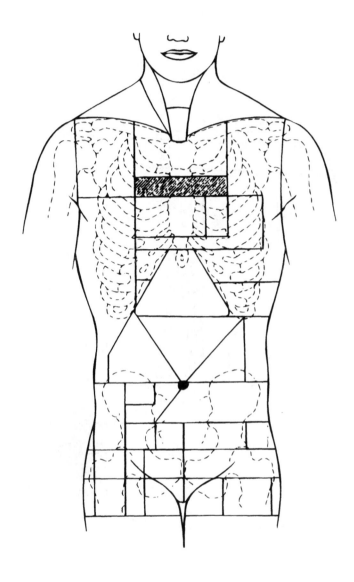

The upper Star of Bethlehem zone on the trunk begins in the second intercostal space, at the width of approximately one hand below the collarbone. The zone ends in the third intercostal space. The zone extends 4 finger widths to the left and right of the midline. The Star of Bethlehem remedy covers the entire navel, including both the inside and the border.

STAR OF BETHLEHEM

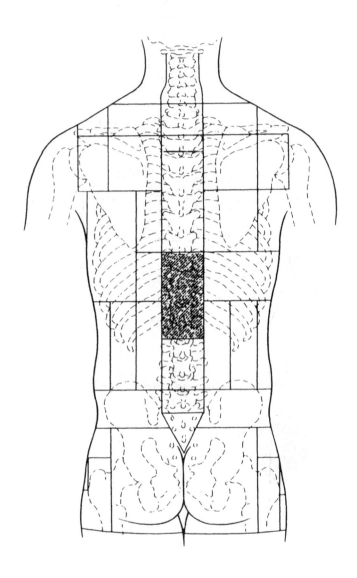

The Star of Bethlehem zone on the back begins at the level of the eighth thoracic vertebra and ends at the level of the first lumbar vertebra. The side borders are 2 finger widths to the left and right of the midline.

Star of Bethlehem

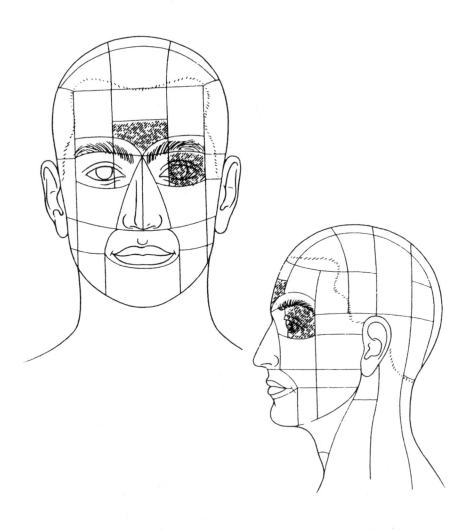

The Star of Bethlehem remedy applies to two zones on the face. The upper zone begins in the middle of the forehead and extends to the point of intersection of the eyebrows. The zone extends 1½ finger widths to either sides of the midline, to the peak of the eyebrows.

The lower zone begins at the lower end of the left eyebrow and ends at the lower edge of the eye socket. The inside border aligns vertically with the inner edge of the iris; the outside border aligns vertically with the end of the eyebrow.

STAR OF BETHLEHEM

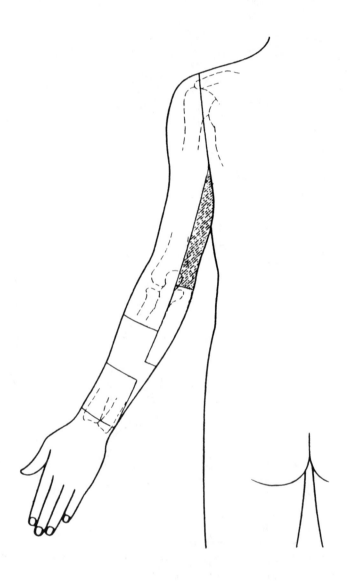

The Star of Bethlehem zone on the left arm begins in the middle of the armpit and ends at the level of the elbow. The front border runs along the inner edge of the biceps muscle; its upper end lies in the axial fold. The back border lies 1 finger width to the side of the elbow and extends upward into the axial fold.

STAR OF BETHLEHEM

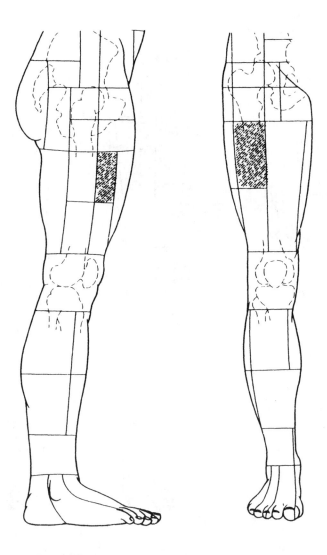

The Star of Bethlehem zone located on the right thigh begins on a horizontal line 1 finger width below the fold of the buttock and ends at a point equidistant between its upper border and a horizontal line 1 finger width above the kneecap. The front border is formed by a vertical line 2 finger widths to the side of the kneecap's right edge. The zone extends 3 finger widths to the back, aligning vertically with the front axial fold.

STAR OF BETHLEHEM

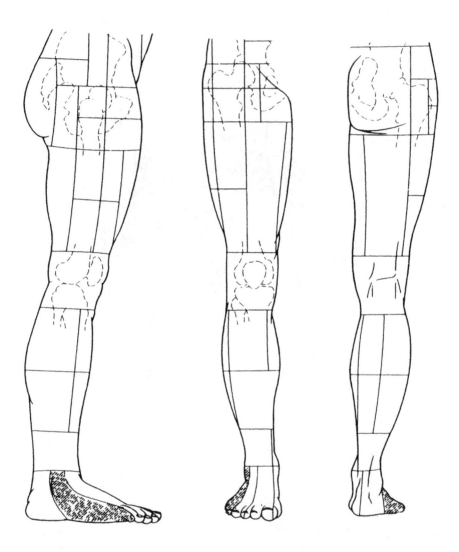

On the outside of the right foot, the Star of Bethlehem zone begins at the top of the outer ankle bone and extends to the little toe. The medial border runs from the front of the outer ankle bone down the foot to the space between the fourth and fifth toes. The lateral border starts behind the outer ankle bone and slopes downward and forward to the bottom of the foot. The inside of the little toe belongs to this zone.

Sweet Chestnut

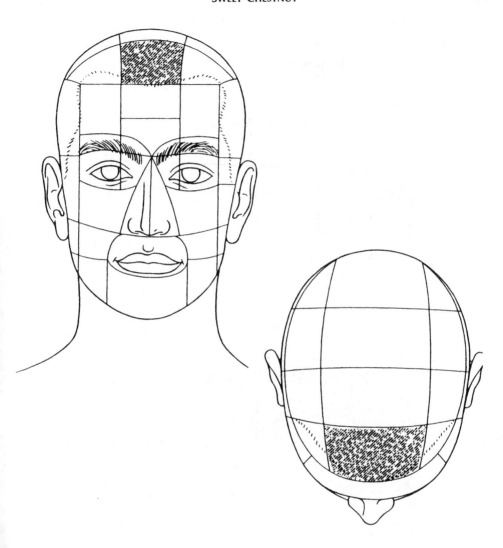

The Sweet Chestnut zone at the head begins at the hairline and ends 3 finger widths behind it. The side borders lie 1½ finger widths to the left and right of the head's midline.

SWEET CHESTNUT

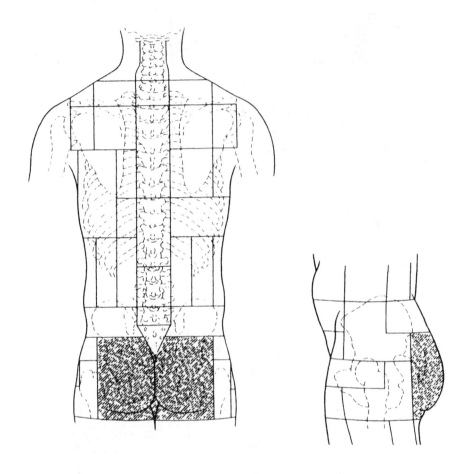

This Sweet Chestnut zone begins at the middle of the sacrum and ends 1 finger width below the fold of the buttocks. (The Pine flower applies to the sacrum itself. See page 166.) The zone extends 2 hand widths to either side, and includes the inner side of the buttocks. The zone ends at a point between the anus and the genitals.

SWEET CHESTNUT

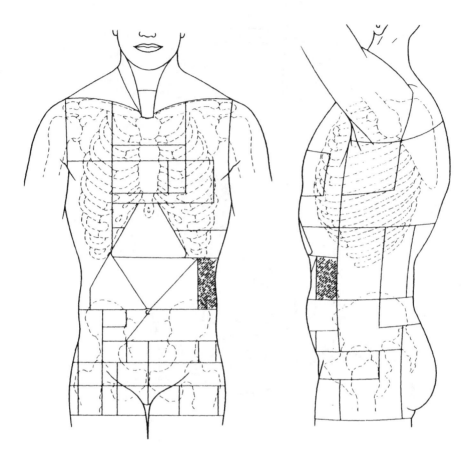

The bottom border of this Sweet Chestnut zone aligns horizontally with the navel, while the upper border sits at the midpoint between the lowest part of the sternum and the navel. The medial border aligns vertically with the left nipple. The lateral border aligns vertically with the front axial fold.

SWEET CHESTNUT

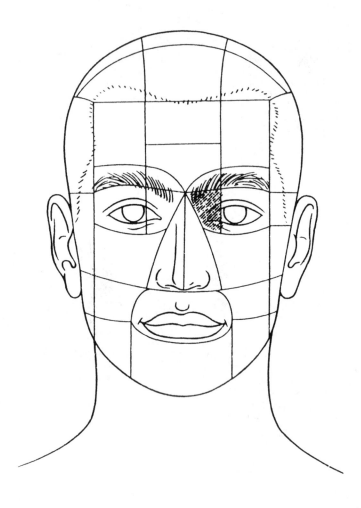

The Sweet Chestnut zone on the face is located in the inside corner of the left eye. Its upper border follows the line of the eyebrow; the lower border is the lower edge of the eye socket. The inside border follows the inner edge of the eye socket. The outside border is marked by a vertical line through the inside edge of the iris.

SWEET CHESTNUT

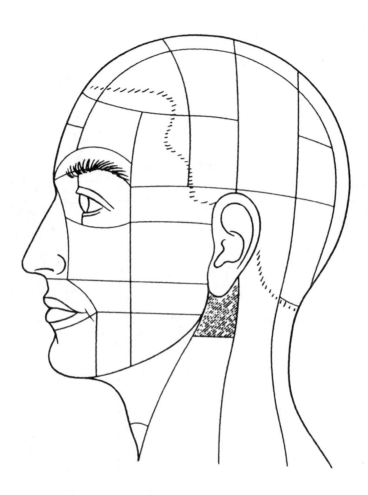

This Sweet Chestnut zone extends from the left ear downward to the level of the jaw. The side borders follow vertically downward from the front and back sides of the ear.

SWEET CHESTNUT

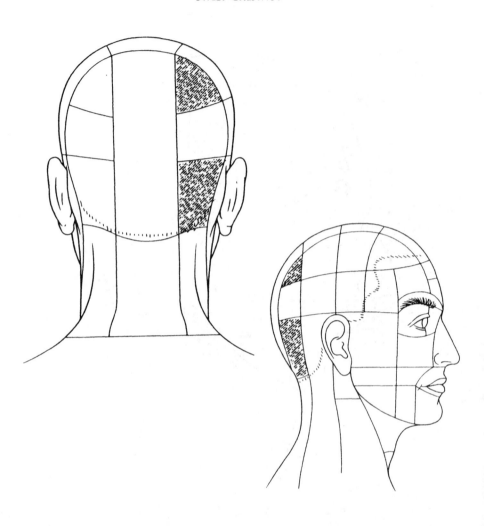

The Sweet Chestnut remedy applies to two zones on the right side of the head. The upper zone begins 3 finger widths behind the crown of the head and extends 3 finger widths backward. The medial border lies 1½ finger widths to the side of the midline.

The lower Sweet Chestnut zone on the head aligns horizontally with the tip of the ear and extends downward to the lower ridge of the skull. The lateral border lies 2 finger widths behind the base of the right ear; the zone extends 3 finger widths toward the back.

SWEET CHESTNUT

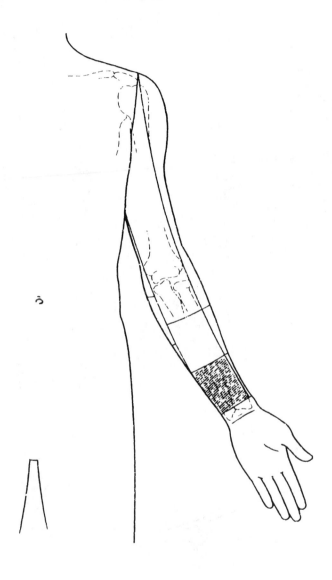

The Sweet Chestnut zone located on the inside of the lower left arm begins 1 finger width above the wrist and extends upward 5 finger widths. The inside border runs along an imaginary line extending from the outside edge of the little finger. The outside border runs along the edge of the radius.

SWEET CHESTNUT

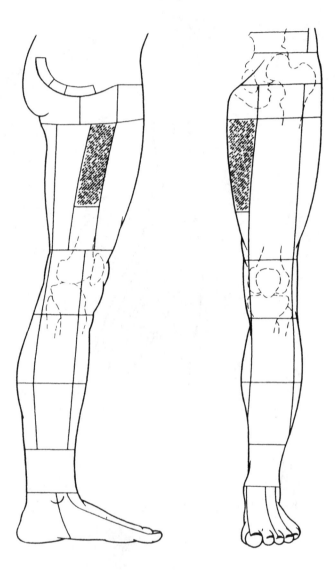

The Sweet Chestnut zone located on the inside of the left thigh begins at a level of 1 finger width below the fold of the buttock and ends 5 finger widths above the kneecap. The inside margin lies 1 finger width to the inside of the kneecap. The zone extends 3 finger widths toward the inside of the thigh.

SWEET CHESTNUT

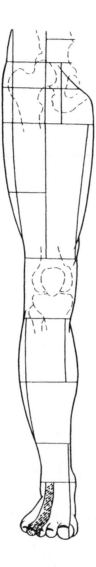

The Sweet Chestnut zone on the right foot begins horizontal to the upper edge of the inside ankle bone and extends downward to the toes. The inside border runs from the middle of the ankle fold to the middle of the middle toe. The outside border begins at the front edge of the inside ankle bone and extends downward to the space between the fourth and fifth toes. The zone ends at the beginning of the sole of the foot.

SWEET CHESTNUT

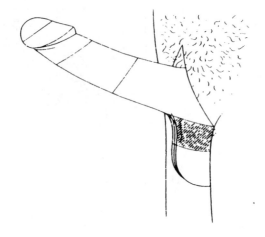

The Sweet Chestnut remedy also applies to the upper half of the left testicle.
The zone begins at the midline and ends at the base of the scrotum.

VERVAIN

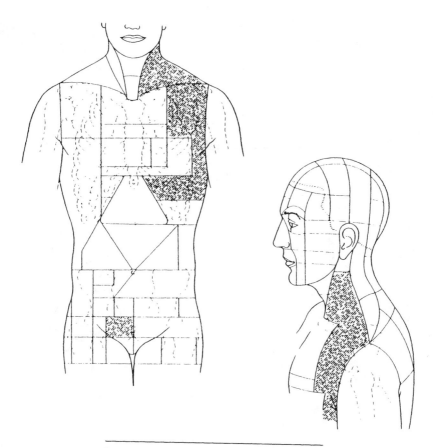

The Vervain remedy covers a large area on the left side of the trunk. The upper zone begins 2 finger widths below the ear and extends downward along the edge of the trapezius muscle to the outer end of the collarbone. The lateral border continues downward from the front axial fold. The border at the front of the neck is formed by the sternocleidomastoid muscle. Up to the level of the third intercostal space, the medial border is located 4 finger widths to the side of midline. From the third to the sixth intercostal space the medial border is 8 finger widths from midline. The medial border continues along the costal arch. The zone ends on a horizontal line 3 finger widths below the lower edge of the sternum.

The lower zone begins one finger width above the upper edge of the pubic bone and ends at the lower edge of the pubic bone. The zone extends 4 finger widths to the right of midline.

VERVAIN

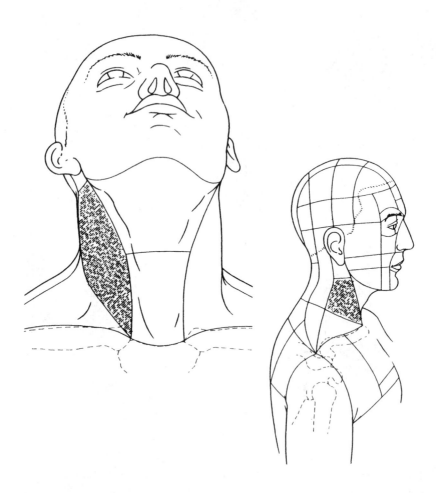

The Vervain zone on the right side of the neck begins 2 finger widths below the right ear, aligning vertically with the back of the ear and extending downward to the base of the neck. The zone runs along the base of the neck to the collarbone. The front border is formed by the ridge of the sterno-cleidomastoid muscle.

VERVAIN

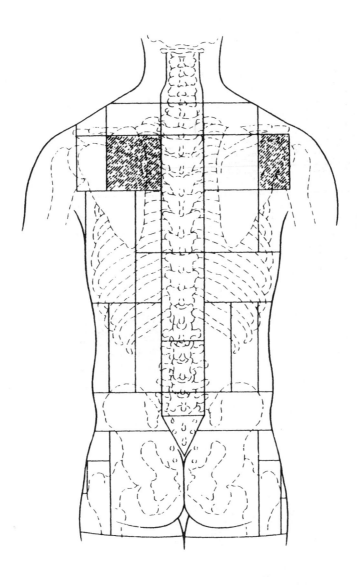

The two Vervain zones on the back begin at the level of the second thoracic vertebra and end at the level of the fifth thoracic vertebra. The left zone begins 2 finger widths from the midline and extends 6 finger widths to the left. The lateral aspect of the right zone aligns vertically with the back axial fold. The zone extends 3 finger widths toward the midline.

VERVAIN

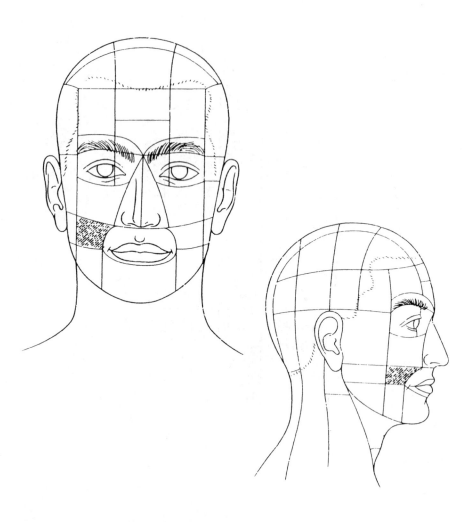

The Vervain zone on the right side of the face aligns horizontally with the bottom of the nose and extends downward to align horizontally with the corner of the mouth. The inside border follows a curved line from the nose to the right corner of the mouth. The outside border aligns vertically with the end of the eyebrow.

VERVAIN

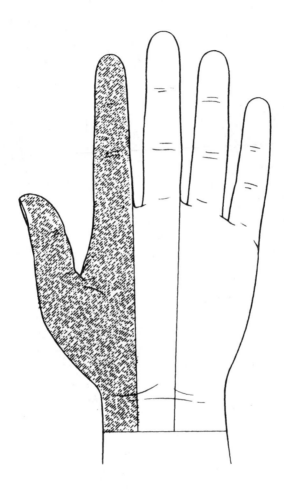

The Vervain zone located on the inside of the left hand extends from 1 finger width above the wrist to the tips of the thumb and index finger. The left border runs from the edge of the wrist to the corner of the thumbnail. The right border begins 1 finger width inside the wrist and extends to the right side of the index finger.

VERVAIN

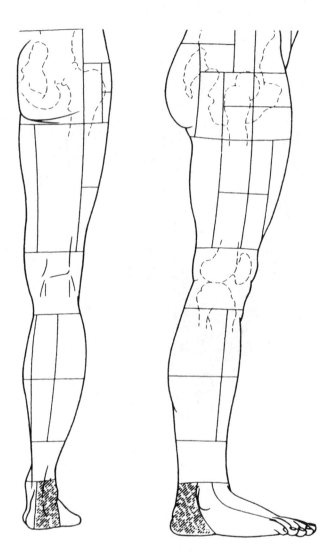

This Vervain zone is located on the right foot in the area of the right outer ankle bone. It begins at the level of the ankle bone's upper edge and ends at the lower edge of the foot. The back border is formed by the Achilles tendon; the front border begins at the back side of the outer ankle bone and runs in a slope toward the front.

VERVAIN

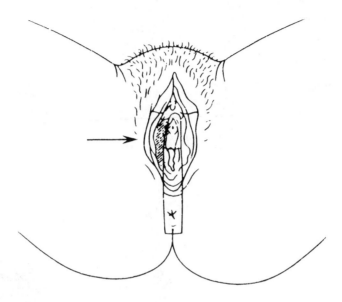

The Vervain remedy covers the inside of the right labia minora.

VINE

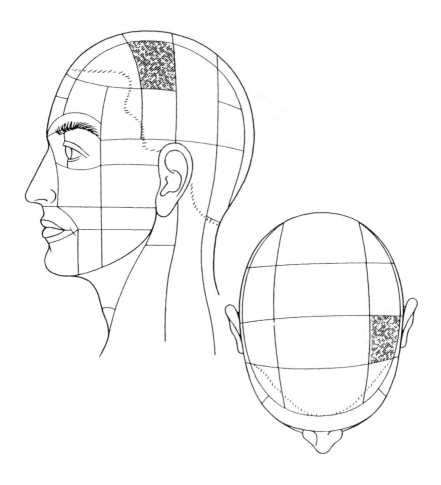

The Vine zone on the left side of the head begins 1½ finger widths to the side of midline and ends 3 finger widths above the tip of the left ear. The back border aligns vertically with the tip of the ear. The zone extends 3 finger widths toward the front.

VINE

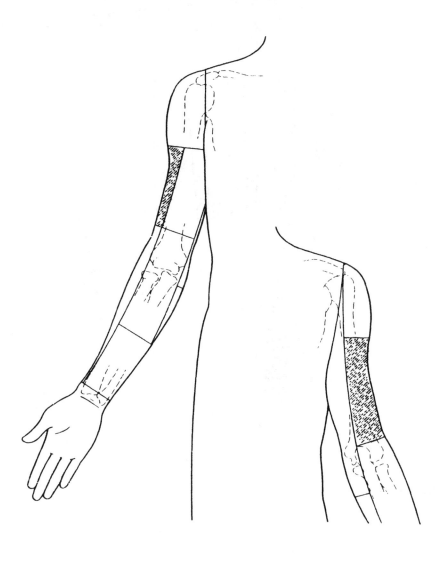

The Vine zone on the right upper arm begins at the level of the axial fold and ends 6 finger widths above the elbow. The back border lies 3 finger widths to the right of the back axial fold. The front border follows the outside edge of the biceps muscle.

VINE

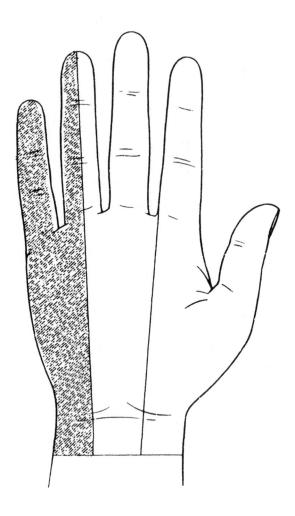

The Vine zone located on the inside of the right hand extends from 1 finger width above the wrist to the tips of the ring and little fingers. The left border runs along the outside edge of the hand to the outside corner of the little fingernail. The border to the right begins 1 finger width to the right of the edge of the wrist and extends upward to the middle of the ring finger.

VINE

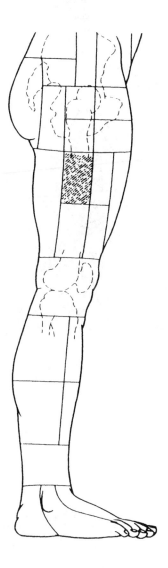

The Vine zone located on the outside of the right thigh begins at the level of 1 finger width below the fold of the buttock and ends midway between this upper border and 1 finger width above the kneecap. The left and right borders of this zone align vertically with the front and back axial folds.

VINE

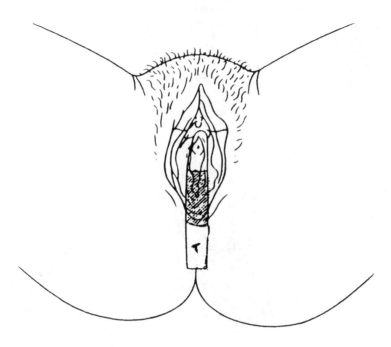

The Vine zone at the genitals begins at the upper margin of the vagina and ends above the anus, at the area where the color of the skin changes from red to the hue of the surrounding skin. The outer borders are formed by the labia minora.

WALNUT

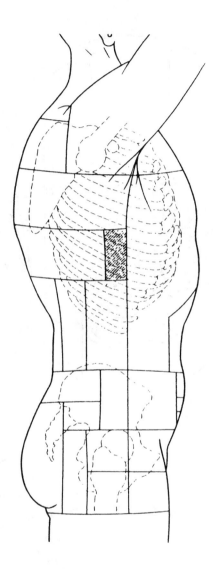

The Walnut zone located on the right side of the body underneath the arm begins at the level of the eighth thoracic vertebra and ends at the level of the eleventh thoracic vertebra. The front border aligns vertically with the front axial fold. The zone extends 2½ finger widths to the back.

WALNUT

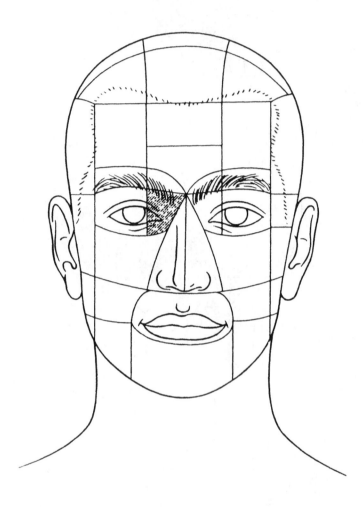

The Walnut zone on the face is located on the inside corner of the right eye. The upper border extends outward horizontal to the midpoint between the eyebrows. The lower border is the lower rim of the eye socket. The interior edge is formed by an extension of the inner eye socket rim upward to the midpoint between the eyebrows. The outer edge aligns vertically with the inside edge of the iris.

WALNUT

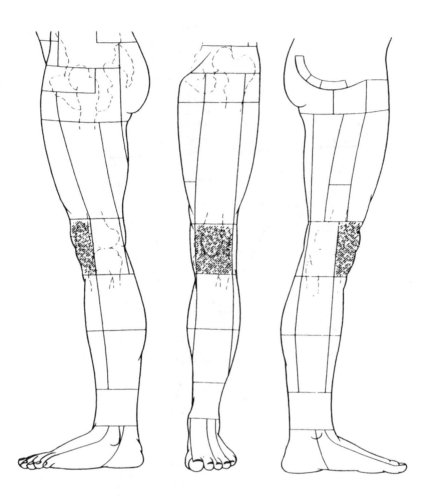

The Walnut zone covering the left kneecap begins 1 finger width above the kneecap and ends 3½ finger widths below the kneecap's lower edge. The borders to the sides are 2½ finger widths to the left and right of the kneecap.

WATER VIOLET

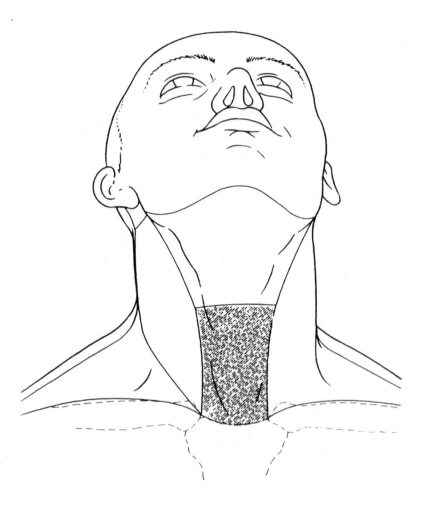

The Water Violet zone on the front of the neck extends from the upper rim of the sternum to the middle of the Adam's apple. The side borders are formed by the inside edges of the two sternocleidomastoid muscles.

WATER VIOLET

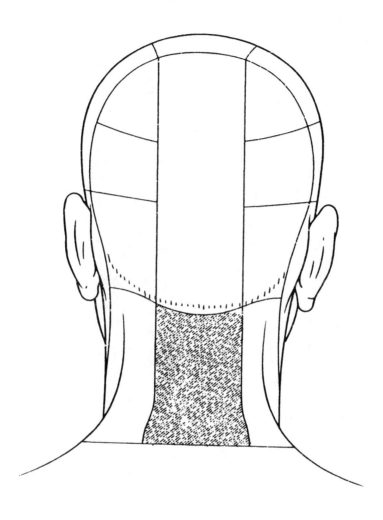

The Water Violet zone on the back of the neck begins at the level of the sixth cervical vertebra and ends at the base of the skull. The borders to the sides are located 1½ finger widths to the left and right of midline.

WATER VIOLET

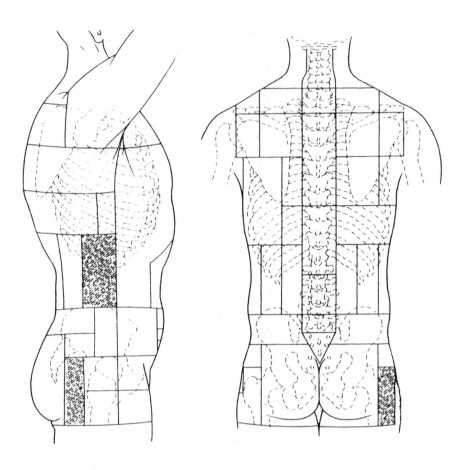

There are two Water Violet zones located on the right side of the body. The upper zone begins at the level of the eleventh thoracic vertebra and ends at the level of the fourth lumbar vertebra. The side borders align vertically with the front and back axial folds.

The lower zone begins at the level of 1 finger width above the pubic bone and ends at the level 1 finger width below the fold of the buttock. The front border aligns vertically with the front axial fold. The zone extends 3 finger widths to the back.

Water Violet

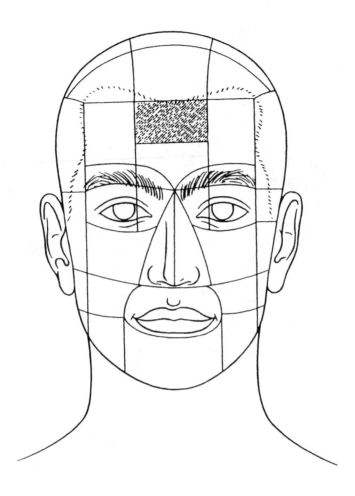

The Water Violet zone on the forehead begins at the hairline and ends midway between the hairline and the intersection of the eyebrows. The outer borders are located 1½ finger widths to the right and left of midline.

WATER VIOLET

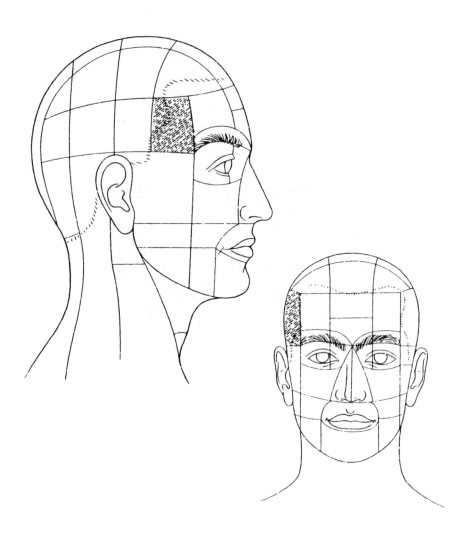

The Water Violet zone on the right side of the head begins at the level of the hairline and ends horizontal to the edge of the eyebrow. The inside border aligns vertically with the edge of the eyebrow. The zone extends 2½ finger widths toward the back.

WATER VIOLET

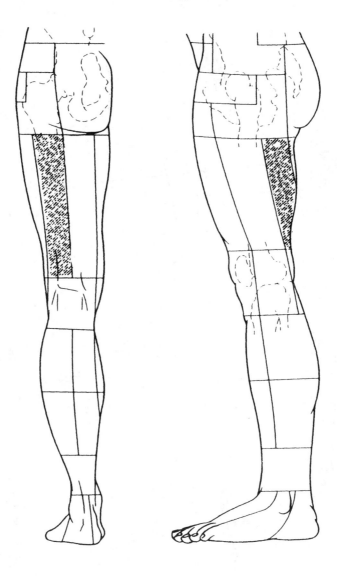

The lateral border of the Water Violet zone located on the back of the left thigh aligns vertically with the back axial fold. The zone extends 2½ finger widths to the right to the middle of the thigh. The upper border lies 1 finger width below the fold of the buttock. The lower border lies 1 finger width above the kneecap.

WATER VIOLET

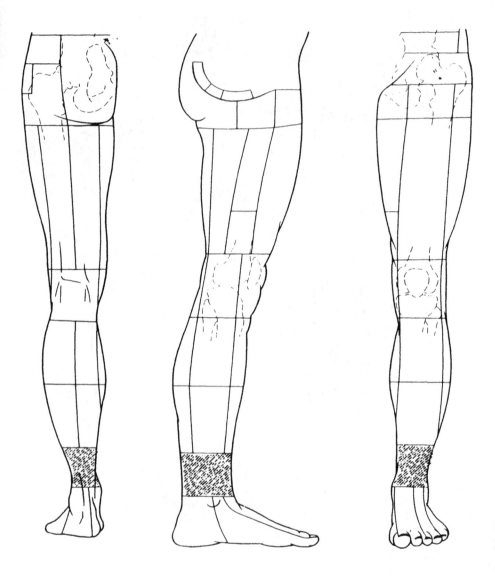

This Water Violet zone encircles the lower part of the left leg. It begins at the level of the ankle bone's upper edge and extends 4 finger widths upward.

WATER VIOLET

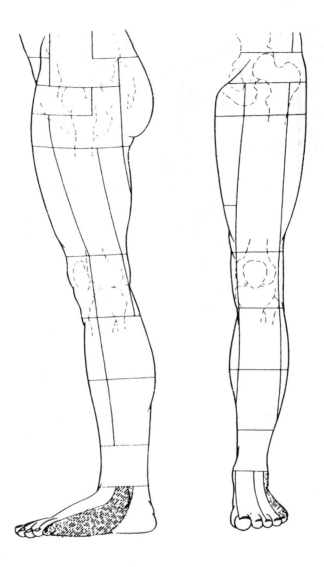

The Water Violet zone located on the left foot begins at the top of the outer ankle bone and continues to the little toe. The front side runs from the front of the outer ankle bone to the space between the fourth and fifth toes. The back border starts behind the ankle bone and slopes toward the sole of the foot. The zone ends at the beginning of the sole of the foot. The inside of the little toe belongs to this zone.

WHITE CHESTNUT

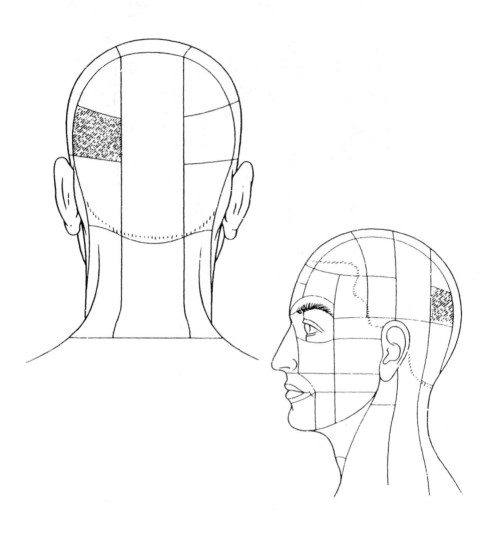

The White Chestnut zone on the left side of the head begins 3 finger widths behind the tip of the left ear and extends 3 finger widths toward the back. The lower border aligns with the tip of the ear. The upper border lies 3 finger widths above this.

White Chestnut

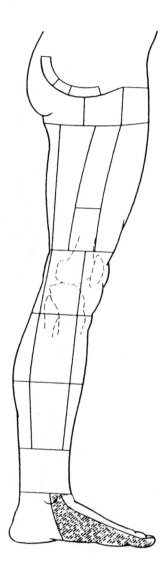

This White Chestnut zone extends from the upper edge of the left inside ankle bone to the lower edge of the left foot. The back border runs from the midpoint of the ankle bone downward in a mild slope toward the sole of the foot. The front border runs from the front edge of the ankle to the inside corner of the big toe.

WHITE CHESTNUT

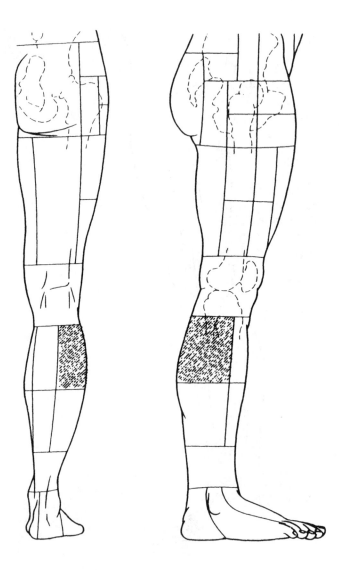

The White Chestnut zone located on the right calf begins 3½ finger widths below the right kneecap and extends 6 finger widths downward. The lateral border lies 2 finger widths to the side of the kneecap; the medial border aligns vertically with the Achilles tendon and the middle of the back of the knee.

WILD OAT

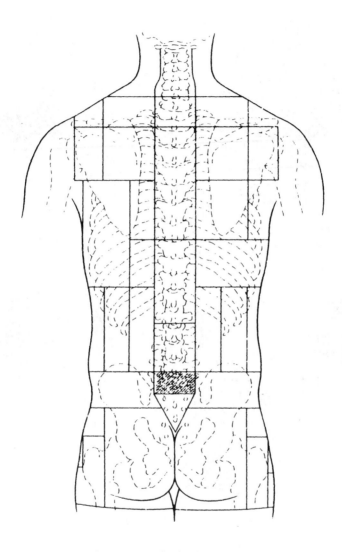

The Wild Oat zone on the back starts at the level of the fourth lumbar vertebra and ends at the upper border of the sacrum. The side borders are located 2 finger widths to the left and right of midline.

WILD OAT

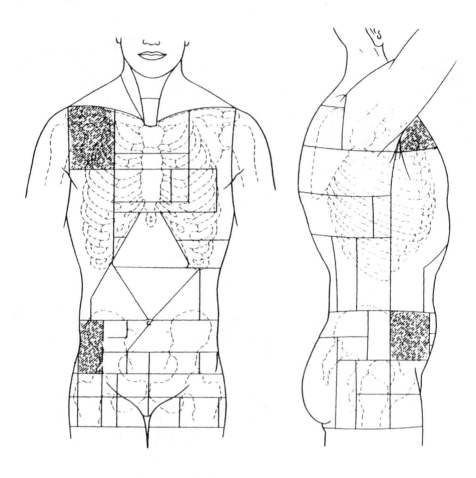

There are two Wild Oat zones on the front of the body. The upper zone begins at the outer half of the right clavicle and ends in the third intercostal space. The medial border is located 4 finger widths to the right of the midline; the lateral border aligns vertically with the axial line. The lower zone begins at the level of the umbilicus and ends 1 finger width above the pubic bone. The medial border aligns vertically with the right nipple; the lateral border aligns vertically with the front axial fold.

Wild Rose

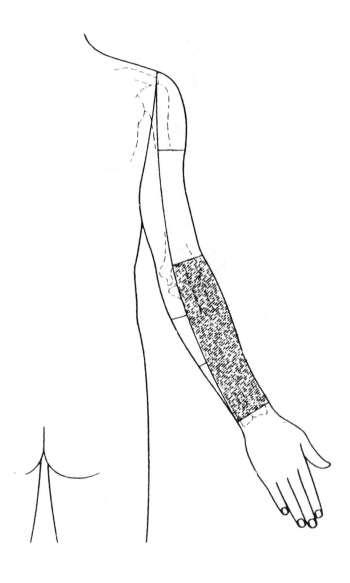

The Wild Rose remedy applies to the upper side of the right forearm. It begins 4 finger widths above the tip of the elbow and ends 1 finger width above the wrist. The thumb-side border runs along the outer edge of the radius and continues upward along the outer edge of the biceps muscle. The border on the little-finger side runs along the outside edge of the ulna to end 1 finger width away from the tip of the elbow.

WILD ROSE

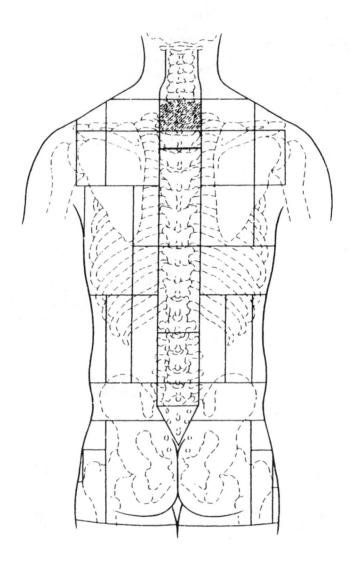

The Wild Rose zone on the back begins at the level of the sixth cervical vertebra and ends at the level of the second thoracic vertebra. The side borders are located 2 finger widths to the left and right of midline.

WILD ROSE

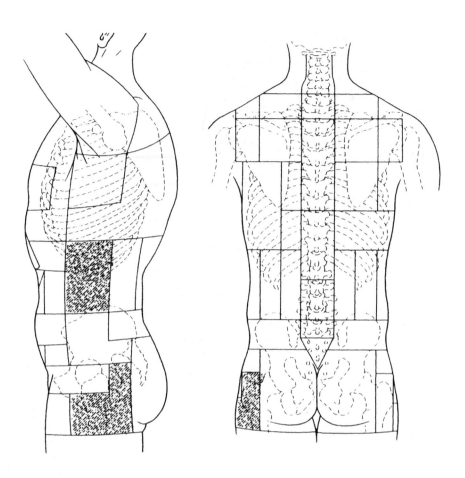

There are two Wild Rose zones located on the left side of the body. The upper zone begins at the level of the eleventh thoracic vertebra and ends at the level of the fourth lumbar vertebra. The side borders align with the front and back axial folds.

The lower zone begins 1 finger width below the fold of the buttock. The front border aligns vertically with the front axial fold. Its upper margin aligns with the lower side of the pubic bone. The zone extends backward to 3 finger widths beyond the vertical line of the back axial fold, the uppermost margin ending 1 finger width above the pubic bone.

WILD ROSE

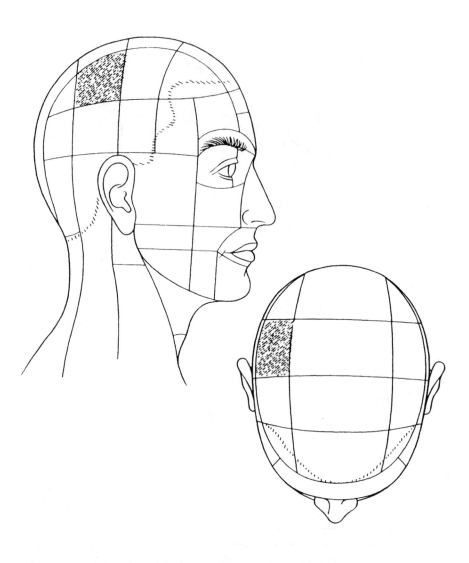

The Wild Rose zone on the right side of the head begins 1½ finger widths to the side of midline and ends 3 finger widths above the tip of the right ear. The front border aligns vertically with the tip of the ear. The zone extends 3 finger widths toward the back.

WILD ROSE

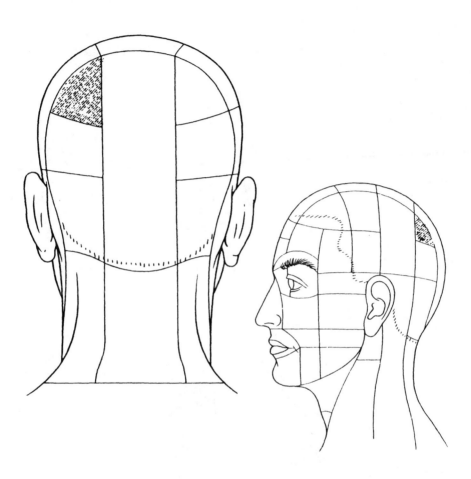

The Wild Rose zone on the left side of the head begins 3 finger widths behind the tip of the left ear and extends 3 finger widths toward the back. The upper border lies 1½ finger widths to the side of midline; the lower border lies 3 finger widths above the tip of the ear.

WILD ROSE

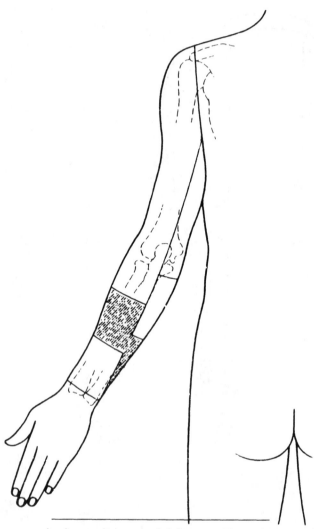

Wild Rose remedy also applies to the left forearm. The upper part of the zone begins 6 finger widths above the wrist and extends 5 finger widths upward. The thumb-side border runs alongside the edge of the radius; the little-finger-side border runs alongside the edge of the ulna.

The lower part of the zone begins on a horizontal line 1 finger width above the wrist and extends 7 finger widths upward. The outer border runs along the edge of the ulna. The inner border runs on a vertical line from the outer edge of the little finger toward the inner fold of the elbow.

WILD ROSE

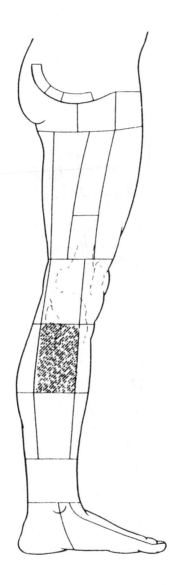

The Wild Rose zone on the left leg begins 3½ finger widths below the left kneecap and extends 6 finger widths downward. The front border lies 2 finger widths to the side of the kneecap. The zone extends 3 finger widths toward the back.

WILD ROSE

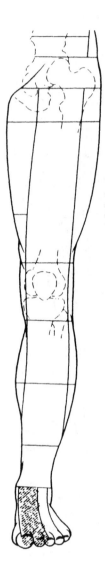

The Wild Rose zone on the left foot begins at the upper edge of the inner ankle bone and continues to the toes. The medial margin runs from the ankle to the outside corner of the big toe. The lateral margin runs down the foot to the midline of the middle toe. The lower border is located at the beginning of the sole of the foot; the insides of the toes belong to this zone.

WILLOW

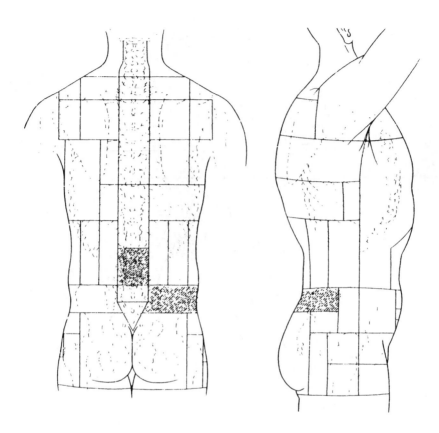

There are two Willow zones on the back. The upper zone begins at the level of the first lumbar vertebra and ends at the level of the fourth lumbar vertebra. The side borders lie 2 finger widths to the left and right of midline.

The lower zone on the right side of the body begins at the level of the fourth lumbar vertebra and extends downward to the midpoint of the sacrum. The inside border is located at the edge of the spinal column, 2 finger widths to the side of midline, and slopes toward the anal fold following the edge of the sacrum (the sacroiliac joint). The zone extends laterally approximately 10 finger widths.

WILLOW

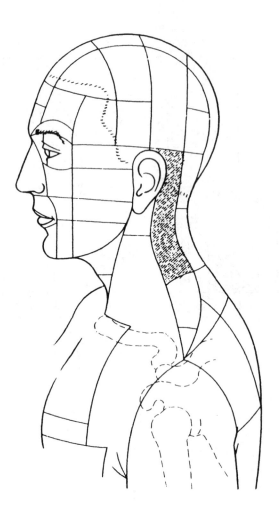

The Willow zone on the left side of the neck begins at the tip of the left ear and ends at the base of the neck. The front border follows the base of the ear, extending downward. The zone extends 2 finger widths to the back.

WILLOW

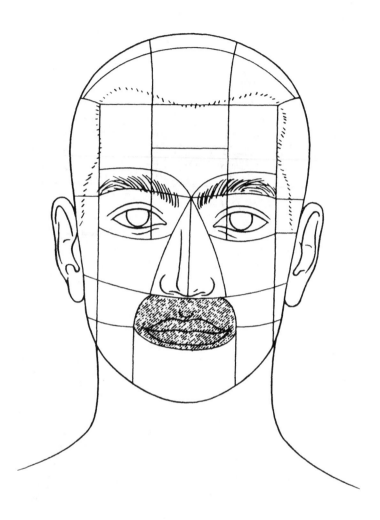

This Willow zone begins at the bottom of the nose and continues in a curved line over the upper lip to the corner of the mouth. The zone ends at the lower rim of the lower lip.

WILLOW

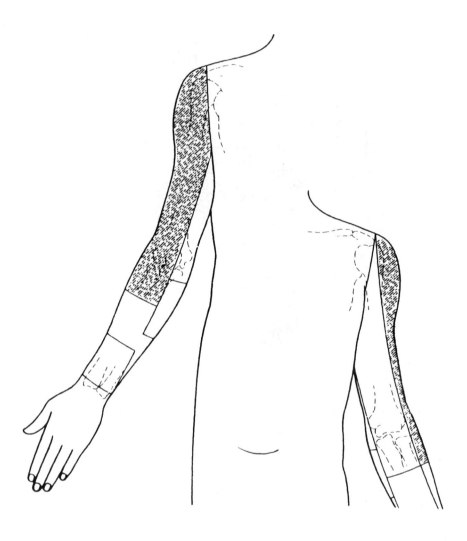

The Willow zone on the left upper arm begins at the acromioclavicular joint, the meeting point of the front and back axial folds. From there the zone extends downward to end 3 finger widths below the tip of the elbow. The back border lies on a line that begins 1 finger width to the side of the tip of the elbow and ends in the back axial fold. The front border runs alongside the outer edge of the biceps muscle.

WILLOW

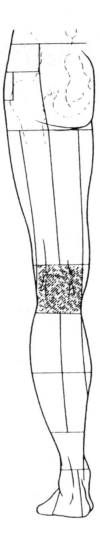

This Willow zone is located at the back of the left knee, extending 2½ finger widths to each side of the midline. The upper border aligns horizontally 1 finger width above the kneecap; the lower border aligns horizontally 3½ finger widths below the kneecap.

APPENDIX I

TOPOGRAPHICAL SUMMARY OF THE BACH FLOWER BODY MAPS

The following illustrations show each skin zone keyed by number to its appropriate Bach Flower remedy. The remedies are listed below in alphabetical order.

1. Agrimony	20. Mimulus
2. Aspen	21. Mustard
3. Beech	22. Oak
4. Centaury	23. Olive
5. Cerato	24. Pine
6. Cherry Plum	25. Red Chestnut
7. Chestnut Bud	26. Rock Rose
8. Chicory	27. Rock Water
9. Clematis	28. Scleranthus
10. Crab Apple	29. Star of Bethlehem
11. Elm	30. Sweet Chestnut
12. Gentian	31. Vervain
13. Gorse	32. Vine
14. Heather	33. Walnut
15. Holly	34. Water Violet
16. Honeysuckle	35. White Chestnut
17. Hornbeam	36. Wild Oat
18. Impatiens	37. Wild Rose
19. Larch	38. Willow

This topographical summary is available as a wall chart from:

D. Münks Verlag, Dohlenweg 16, D-40668 Meerbusch
Phone: (02150) 32 12
Fax: (02150) 66 13

Head

TOP

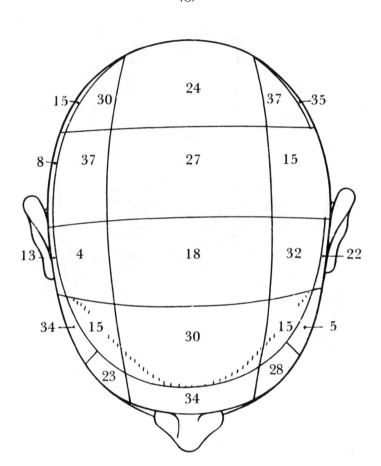

Head

ANTERIOR

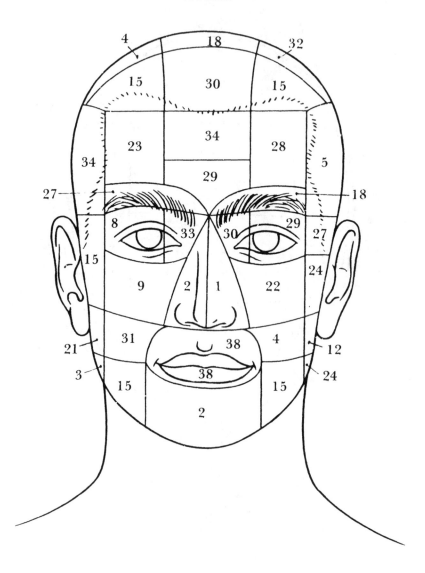

HEAD

RIGHT SIDE

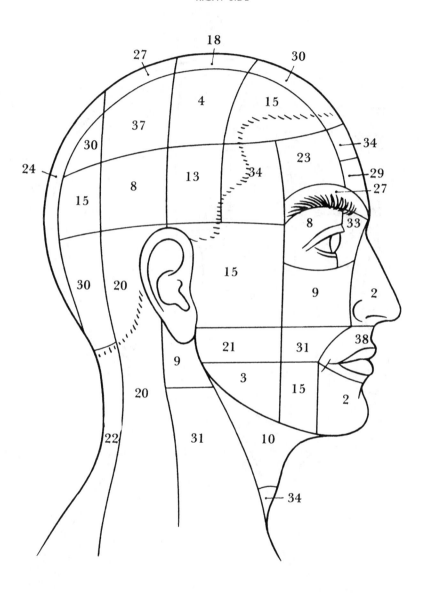

HEAD

LEFT SIDE

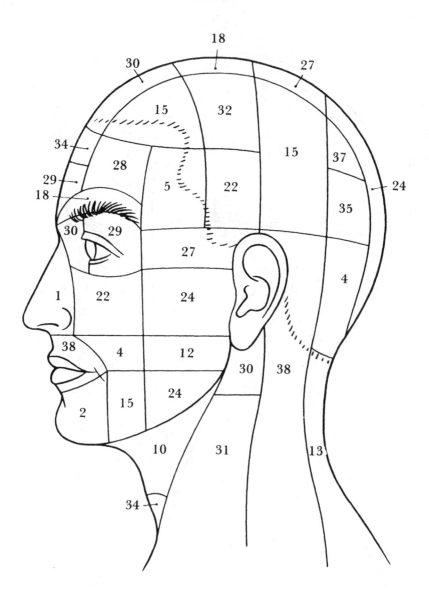

Head

POSTERIOR

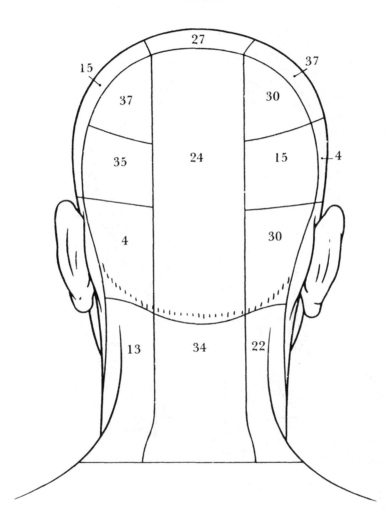

NECK

ANTERIOR

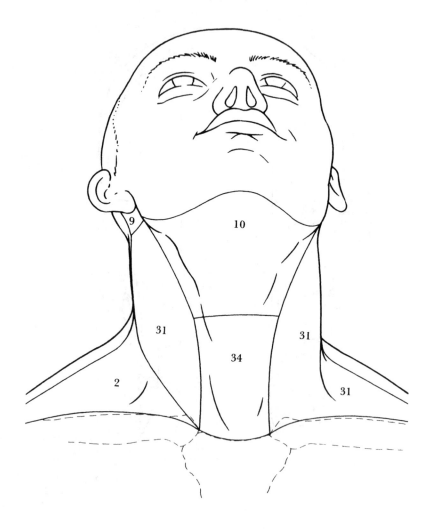

HEAD AND RIGHT SOULDER

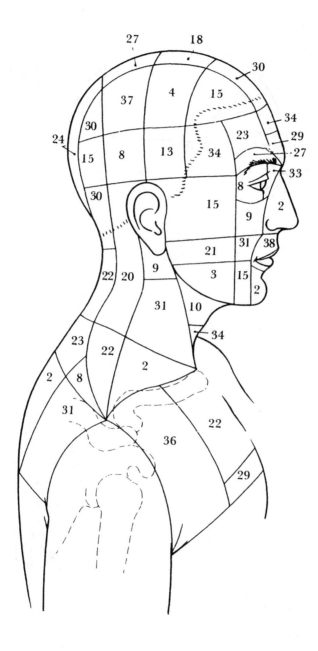

Head and Left Sholder

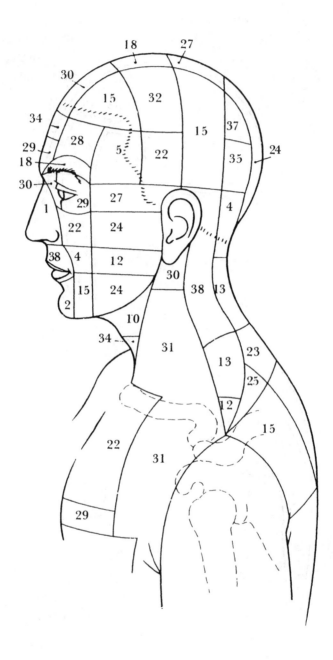

TRUNK

ANTERIOR

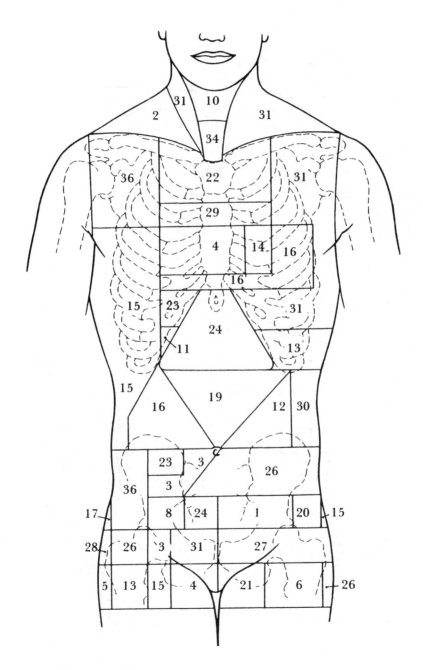

TRUNK

POSTERIOR

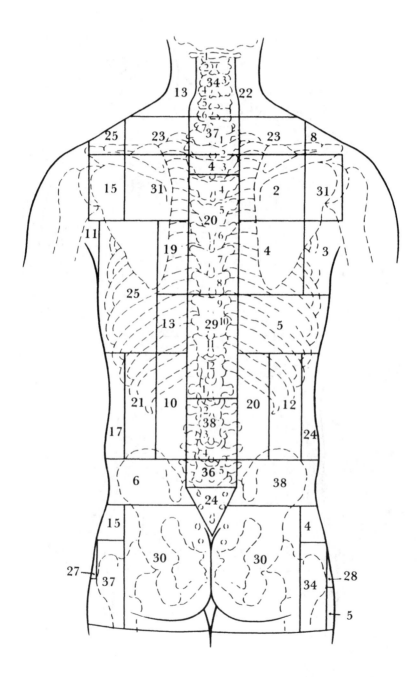

TRUNK

RIGHT SIDE

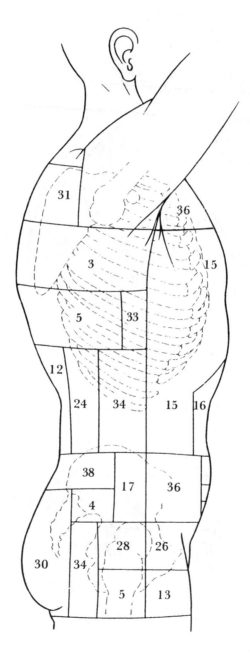

TRUNK

LEFT SIDE

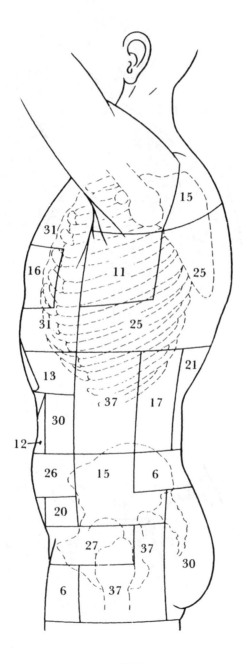

GENITALS

FEMALE

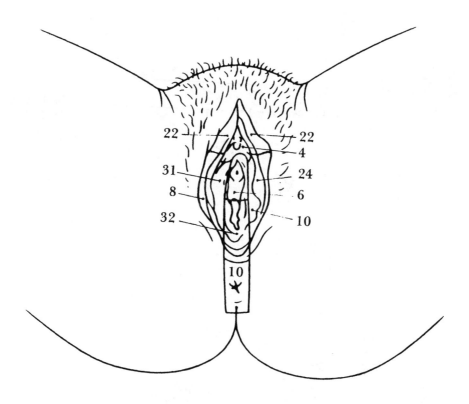

Genitals

MALE

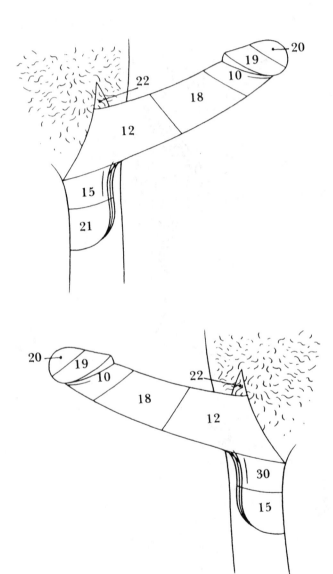

Legs

Anterior

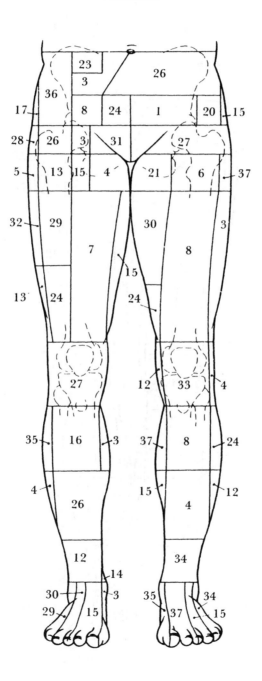

LEGS

POSTERIOR

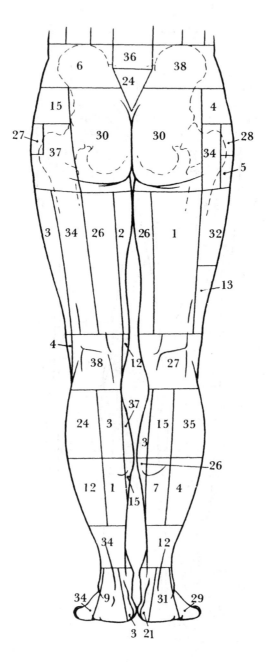

Right Leg

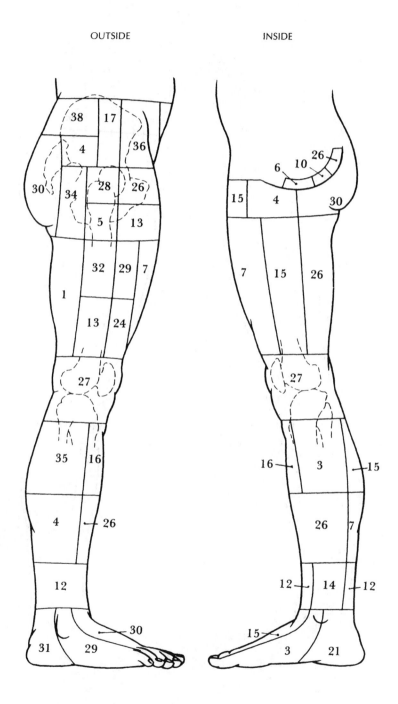

OUTSIDE

INSIDE

265

LEFT LEG

INSIDE   OUTSIDE

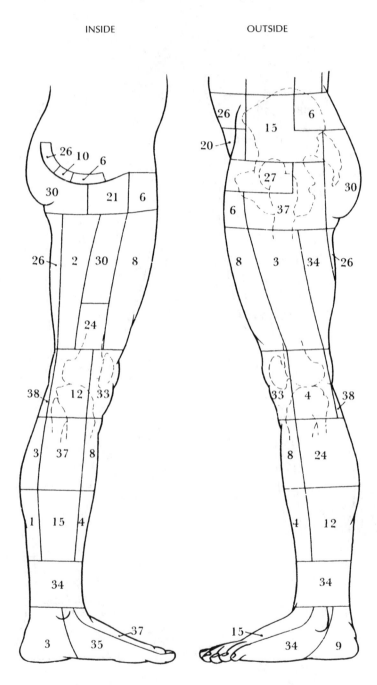

SOLE OF THE FOOT

RIGHT

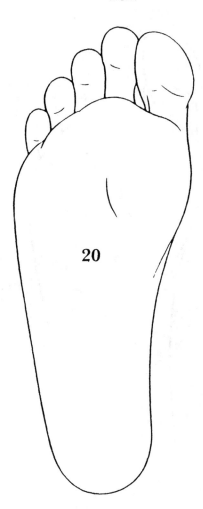

20

SOLE OF THE FOOT

LEFT

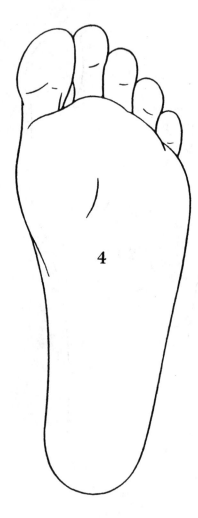

4

Right Arm

FROM BEHIND

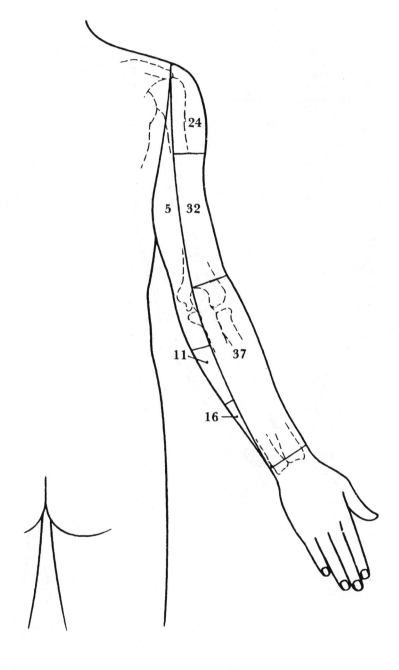

Right Arm

FROM THE FRONT

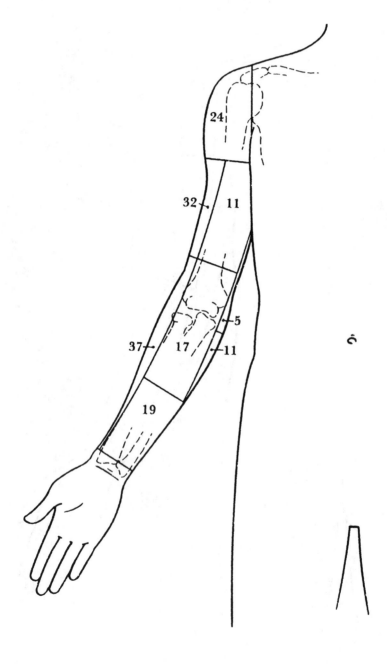

Left Arm

From Behind

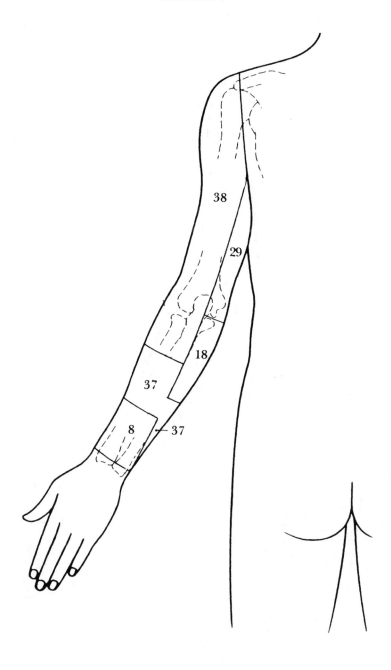

LEFT ARM

FROM THE FRONT

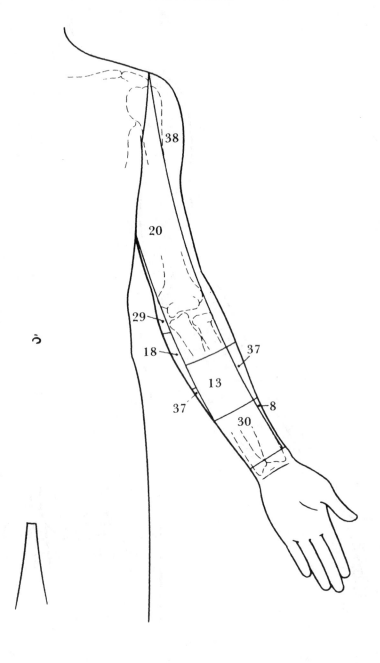

RIGHT HAND

POSTERIOR

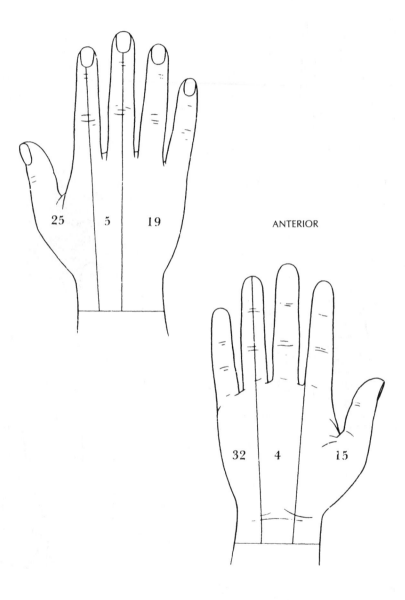

ANTERIOR

LEFT HAND

POSTERIOR

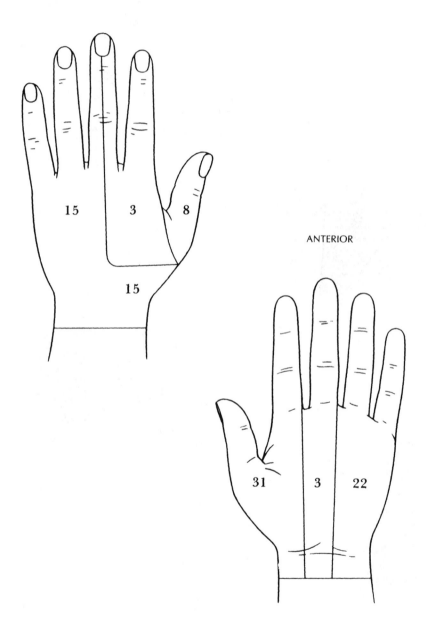

ANTERIOR

APPENDIX II

THE AURA

Knowledge about the aura, the energy field that surrounds each living thing, is as old as humanity itself. The aura is discussed in the oldest known scriptures, such as the Vedas and the Egyptian Pyramid Texts, sometimes in great detail. For thousands of years Indian yogis have meditated on the energy centers of the aura, which they call the *chakras*. The German mystic Johann Georg Gichtel, a pupil of Jakob Boehme, described those energy centers in his book *Theosophia Practica,* written in 1696. A drawing of Gichtel's that shows the location of the chakras in the body was added to this work posthumously. Systematic research to examine these energy fields was subsequently undertaken by the German Baron Dr. Karl von Reichenbach (1788–1869). In the late nineteenth century, the publications of the founder of the Theosophical Society, H. P. Blavatsky, and her successors Annie Besant and Alice Bailey introduced that so-called "secret knowledge" to the broader public for the first time.

Through anthroposophical medicine, founded by Rudolf Steiner, knowledge of the aura was introduced into naturopathic medicine. The files of a pharmaceutical company founded by Steiner show plants surrounded by an aura.

In his book *The Visible and Invisible Man* published in German in 1964, C. W. Leadbeater exhibited paintings of auras that had been created by artists under the supervision of psychics.

Around the turn of the century the Russian couple Semjon and Walentina Kirlian succeeded in making the phenomena of the aura visible for the first time. Their method was based on the principle that changes in the aura are connected with changes of resistance on the skin. The intensity of the electrical discharge depends on the resistance of the skin, which thereby makes it possible to make the aura indirectly visible as a sort of reflection. The images generated by Kirlian photography were quite similar to the descriptions of auras by psychics.

During the parapsychology boom in the 1960s, Kirlian photography was investigated more thoroughly. It was then recognized that changes in the aura caused by external situations were made visible through Kirlian photography, thus rendering valuable deductions about the aura. If the aura collapsed at a certain location, the energetic discharge would also be missing. When the aura was distended at a certain point, a bigger reflection could be seen in the photograph. The German naturopath Peter Mandel discovered that the reflection in Kirlian photographs corresponds with the energy of the acupuncture meridians that the Chinese call chi.

What exactly is the aura? The best way to describe it is a kind of energy field that surrounds the human body, similar to magnetic fields that surround a magnet rod. It looks like a shining egg whose interior is the physical body. Its expansion is the widest in times of well-being and in conjunction with great vitality. When the body is weakened, as is the case during an illness or as the result of too much work, the aura will decrease in size, depending on the amount of energy one has. A few days before death the energy field of the body collapses almost completely and extends only a half inch to an inch beyond the body.

The colors of one's aura reflect one's emotions and are constantly changing, depending on the state of mind. Dark colors indicate lower feelings and instincts, while light colors show noble character traits such as love, peacefulness, compassion, and spirituality. A mild rose color, for example, indicates compassionate love, while anger reveals itself in a scarlet red to dark or dirty color scale. Hate becomes visible in the form of dense dark clouds that run through the aura and virtually wrap around the body.

There is constant movement in the aura depending on the intensity of the emotions. Surging emotions show themselves as rotating whirls, a feeling of fear as a trembling of the aura, and rage as flashes that shoot out of the aura and sometimes even hit the person who has provoked the rage. In this way anger can literally hurt another.

The ability to see the aura is inherent. Small children are often able to see it, but if they talk to adults about it, they are often misunderstood. Their psychic observations are brushed away as infantile fantasies, their stories relegated to the realm of fairy tales. Since their abilities are not taken seriously and sometimes even cause them problems, such talents usually become stunted at an early age.

In his book *The Boy with Bright Eyes*, Cyril Scott published the diary of a psychic child. When the boy began his diary, he did not know that the people in his surroundings were not able to see "the lights." Therefore, he naively told others about them and was stunned by their reactions, which for him did not make sense at all. The following exerpt shows the difficulties he encountered.

> After Mom had told Dad everything about Mrs. Aldrige, I asked Mom
> why her lights [aura] always turn more blue when she is in church. Her
> answer was, "Is something wrong with your eyes?"
>
> Why didn't Mom answer my question? I would like to know why
> there is so much yellow around Dad's head, almost like dandelions, and
> only blue around Mother's head. When she gives me a hug her lights
> turn pink.
>
> I would like to know why Mildred's lights are in such a turmoil and
> look like a dirty egg. When I told her about it she said: "Oh, just shut
> up, you are crazy."[11]

The boy was examined by an ophthalmologist, who could not find anything wrong with his eyes. An allopathic doctor also could not find anything
wrong with him but wrote him a prescription "just in case." When consulted,
a homeopathic doctor immediately took him off the medicine. Later in the
boy's diary we can read about the homeopathic prescription: "Nevertheless,
the new doctor recommended a change of climate and water applications at
the ocean. It is almost unnecessary to mention that it did not cure my psychic
abilities."[12]

Similar things happened to Lea Sanders when as a little girl she asked,
"Grandma, why are all the colors so beautiful?" "Don't talk about rainbows
around people, child. Nobody else sees them and you just insult people."[13]

If such children meet a person who knows about these matters and can
even train them, the chance exists that their abilities can be preserved beyond
childhood. The boy in Cyril Scott's book found his teacher to be such a
person. He writes in his diary: "Mr. Pattmore found out that the lights I see
are called *the aura* and he taught me to spell the word. During break time we
talked a lot about auras. He seemed to like this topic since he asked me many
questions. I told him that the aura of some people can be compared with a
dirty mass, while other people are surrounded with beautiful light-colored
auras. Then there are people whose aura suddenly stops [meaning the aura
has a clear border], like the one of my mom, while the outer edge of other
people's fades away sort of like a cloud."[14]

Over time these children learn to interpret the colors they see and to
understand people with their "first sight." Lea Sanders writes:

> Uncle Woody, who liked to paint and draw, was green. The adults said
> he was a creative person and so I learned that the nice pine green
> indicates that people like to create something. There were also other
> green people like Uncle Wayne, who always had money problems. His

green was between green and brown and I did not like this color very much, although I liked my uncle very much.

The rainbow of Grandma was the most beautiful one of all. She had lots of the creative green, like the one of Uncle Woody. . . . When she wrote her poems, which she did often, the green was flowing all around Grandma onto the floor.

Grandpa had more blue than anybody else in the family. He thought that everything needed to be done in a certain way and if this did not happen his rainbow changed color and became all red and Grandma said, "Well John, think about it one more time before you get too mad." And so I learned rather quickly that red stood for anger. It was an unpleasant feeling if somebody was mad or unhappy. But on Sunday when the neighbors came to visit in their Sunday clothes and were sitting in the living room, Grandpa talked about how everybody should help one another and the soft blue colors were flowing out of his heart without restraint.[15]

Notes

1. Dr. Edward Bach, *Gesammelte Werke** (Grafing: Aquamarin Verlag, 1988), 31. Source: Lecture 78 in Wallingford.
2. Ibid., 61. Source: *The Twelve Healers.*
3. Ibid., 77. Source: *The Twelve Healers.*
4. Nora Weeks, *The Medical Discoveries of Edward Bach, Physician* (Saffron Walden: C. W. Daniels, 1988), 80.
5. Dr. Edward Bach, *Gesammelte Werke*, 149. Source: *Ye Suffer from Yourselves*, in Gregory Vlamis, *Bach Flower Remedies to the Rescue* (Rochester, Vt.: Healing Arts Press, 1990).
6. Ibid., 41. Source: Letter to the Naturopathic Society, 1934.
7. Ibid., 53. Source: Letters and Other Diverse Scripts.
8. Nora Weeks, 129.
9. Ibid., 105.
10. Dr. Edward Bach and Jens-Erik R. Petersen, *Heile dich selbst mit den Bach-Blüten* (Munich: Droemersche Verlagsanstalt Th. Knaur Nachf., 1988, 133.
11. Cyril Scott, *Der Junge mit den lichten Augen* (Grafing: Aquamarin Verlag, 1984), 26.
12. Ibid., 28.
13. Lea Sanders, *Die Farben deiner Aura* (Munich: Goldmann Verlag, 1989), 13.
14. Cyril Scott, 79.
15. Lea Sanders, 14, 16.

---

* *Collected Works*. Because there is no English version of Edward Bach's *Collected Works*, an English source for each reference has been provided as well.

Resources for Bach Flower Remedies

The original Bach Flower Remedies are still collected at the same sites used by Edward Bach and are prepared according to his method. These original flower essences can be purchased individually or as a complete set from the following suppliers:

North America

Nelson Bach USA
100 Research Drive
Wilmington, MA 01887
Phone: (508) 988-3833
Fax: (508) 988-0233

England

Bach Flower Remedies Ltd.
Dr. Edward Bach Centre
Mount Vernon
Sotwell, Wallingford
Oxfordshire OX10 0PZ
Phone: (01491) 834678
Fax: (01491) 825022
E-mail: centre@bachcentre.com

Australia

Martin & Pleasance
P.O. Box 2054
Richmond
Victoria 3121
Phone: 942-77422
Fax: 942-88431

FURTHER READING

The Bach Flower Remedies. New Canaan, Conn.: Keats, 1977. Includes *Heal Thyself* and *The Twelve Healers and Other Remedies* by Edward Bach, and *The Bach Remedies Repertory* by F. J. Wheeler.

Barnard, Julian. *The Guide to the Bach Flower Remedies.* Saffron Walden, Essex: Daniel, 1971.

Chancellor, Philip. *The Handbook of the Bach Flower Remedies.* New Canaan, Conn.: Keats, 1980.

Damian, Peter. *The Twelve Healers of the Zodiac: The Astrology Handbook of the Bach Flower Remedies.* York Beach, Me.: Weiser, 1986.

Krämer, Dietmar. *New Bach Flower Therapies.* Rochester, Vt.: Healing Arts Press, 1995.

Scheffer, Mechthild. *Bach Flower Therapy: Theory and Practice.* Rochester, Vt.: Healing Arts Press, 1988.

———. *Mastering Bach Flower Therapies.* Rochester, Vt.: Healing Arts Press, 1996.

Vlamis, Gregory. *Bach Flower Remedies to the Rescue.* Rochester, Vt.: Healing Arts Press, 1990.

Weeks, Nora. *The Medical Discoveries of Edward Bach, Physician.* New Canaan, Conn.: Keats, 1979.

INDEX

BOOKS OF RELATED INTEREST

New Bach Flower Therapies
Healing the Emotional and Spiritual Causes of Illness
by Dietmar Krämer

Bach Flower Essences and Chinese Medicine
by Pablo Noriega
Translated by Loey Colebeck

Bach Flower Therapy
Theory and Practice
by Mechthild Scheffer

The Encyclopedia of Bach Flower Therapy
by Mechthild Scheffer

Bach Flowers for Crisis Care
Remedies for Emotional and Psychological Well-being
by Mechthild Scheffer

Advanced Bach Flower Therapy
A Scientific Approach to Diagnosis and Treatment
by Götz Blome, M.D.

Bach Flower Remedies for Children
A Parents' Guide
by Barbara Mazzarella

The Healing Intelligence of Essential Oils
The Science of Advanced Aromatherapy
by Kurt Schnaubelt, Ph.D.

Inner Traditions • Bear & Company
P.O. Box 388
Rochester, VT 05767
1-800-246-8648
www.InnerTraditions.com

Or contact your local bookseller